PRACTICE MANAGEMENT

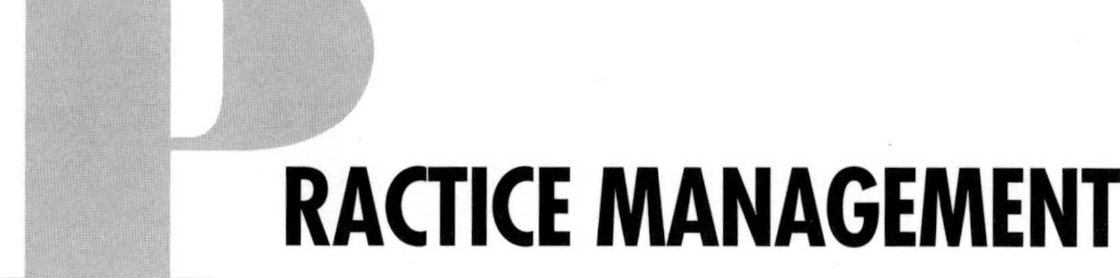

PRACTICE MANAGEMENT

CUMULATIVE INDEX FOR TEXTBOOK OF OPHTHALMOLOGY, VOLS. 1–10

STEPHEN A. KAMENETZKY, MD
Associate Professor of Clinical Ophthalmology
 and Visual Sciences
Washington University School of Medicine
St. Louis, MO

VOLUME 10

TEXTBOOK OF OPHTHALMOLOGY

EDITED BY

STEVEN M. PODOS, MD, FACS
Professor and Chairman
Department of Ophthalmology
Mt. Sinai School of Medicine
New York, NY

MYRON YANOFF, MD, FACS
Professor and Chairman
Department of Ophthalmology
Hahnemann University
Philadelphia, PA

Mosby

London St. Louis Baltimore Boston Chicago Philadelphia Sydney Toronto

For full details of all Mosby-Year Book Europe Ltd. titles, please write to
Mosby-Year Book Europe Ltd., Brook House, 2-16 Torrington Place, London WC1E 7LT, England.

LIBRARY OF CONGRESS CATALOGING-IN-PUBLICATION DATA
(Revised for volume 8)

Textbook of ophthalmology.

Includes bibliographical references and indexes.

1. Ophthalmology. I. Podos, Steven M. II. Yanoff, Myron.
RE46.T26 1991   617.7   91-34425
ISBN ISBN: 1-56375-095-3
ISBN Set: 0-397-44692-6

BRITISH LIBRARY CATALOGUING-IN-PUBLICATION DATA:
A catalogue record for this book is available from the British Library.

ISBN Volume 10: 1-56375-095-3
ISBN Set: 0-397-44692-6

10 9 8 7 6 5 4 3 2 1

Project Manager: LEAH KENNEDY
Art Director and Cover Design: KATHRYN GREENSLADE
Interior Design and Layout: IRINA KOGAN, ENRIQUE SEVILLA
Illustration Director: CAROL KALAFATIC
Illustrator: NICHOLAS GUARRACINO

Produced by Grafos SA
Printed and bound in Spain

EDITORS' DEDICATION

For Dr. Mark A. Podos, my father,
and Dr. Abraham Podos, his father,
my forebearers in eye care.

—SMP

For Jacob Yanoff, MD, the greatest teacher
I have ever known.

—MY

AUTHOR'S DEDICATION

To Phyllis, Andy, and Brian, with love for their unwavering
support despite the endless hours I spent away from them
during the creation of this volume. We did it!

EDITORS' PREFACE

STEVEN M. PODOS, MD, FACS
DEPARTMENT OF
OPHTHALMOLOGY
MT. SINAI SCHOOL OF MEDICINE
NEW YORK, NY

MYRON YANOFF, MD, FACS
DEPARTMENT OF
OPHTHALMOLOGY
HAHNEMANN UNIVERSITY
PHILADELPHIA, PA

As we approach the twenty-first century, it is apparent that the half-life of medical knowledge is continuing to shrink and the amount of current dogma is continuing to expand. Packaging today's relevant ophthalmic knowledge is a difficult chore, yet one that periodically demands doing. Every editor or author desires to accomplish this task in a new and unique fashion. This ten-volume series represents our vision of a *Textbook of Ophthalmology* for the 1990s: one that integrates the basic visual science and clinical information of each subspecialty in a separate volume that is edited or written by noted basic scientists and clinicians; one that is manageable, readable, and affordable for the ophthalmic expert as well as the neophyte; and one that contains original diagrams, figures, and photographs—all in full color—designed to depict the necessary knowledge we hope to impart.

We are grateful to our associate editors and authors for sharing their superb expertise in the compilation of this unique ophthalmic resourse, to our assistants Barbara Zoldessy and Carolyn Lotka for their unstinting efforts in organizing and coordinating this project, and to our wives Wendy Donn Podos and Karin L. Yanoff for their continued patience and encouragement throughout the many phases of this endeavor.

AUTHOR'S PREFACE

STEPHEN A. KAMENETZKY, MD
ST. LOUIS, MO

This book, derived from a series of seminars presented at Academy meetings, is intended to be slightly different from most other volumes on practice management. It does cover all of the standard topics, including personnel matters, billing and bookkeeping, third party payers, computers, malpractice, and risk management. However, the coverage is intended to be ophthalmology-specific, with particular emphasis on common office practice problems and how to avoid or correct them. There are not many books currently available written from this point of view, and I hope that this will make it especially useful.

This volume is primarily intended for residents and new practitioners, although I am sure anyone reading it will be able to pick up a few pointers. It is mostly written from the viewpoint of a solo practitioner or small group, and will probably be of greater value to ophthalmologists thus organized. On the other hand, the section on malpractice and risk management applies to all ophthalmic practices regardless of size.

What I hope will make this volume unique is the inclusion of sections of the ethical and socioeconomic problems that affect every one of us in ophthalmology today. Ethical dilemmas are presented in a way that I hope makes them relevant to many of the difficult situations we all encounter daily. Socioeconomic issues are discussed not only from the point of view of an ophthalmologist in practice but also according to the views of industry, insurers, and the federal and state governments. General liability problems are considered along with medical malpractice concerns because both are similar in many ways and both impact on the development of much of the technology we use today.

These topics were included for a specific reason: the need for physicians to be much more familiar with the general problems related to the economy, insurers, and government than they have been. Formerly, money for health care was plentiful, patients could choose their own physicians, and industry (the primary payer for health care along with the federal government) paid little attention to its own costs. The rapid escalation of health care expenditures and the large federal government budget deficit have ended all this. Different forms of health care delivery are being implemented and others are being proposed. Both trends will have an important impact on all practitioners for many years to come.

To function in the future, ophthalmologists will need to be familiar with all of these problems and how they will affect reimbursement considerations. Government intrusion, in particular, will be come more pervasive and complex. The pertinent chapter in this volume will be helpful; however, because the information is changing rapidly (see Addendum), continued attention will be required. It is hoped that the material presented will stimulate interest in this area and serve as good background for future study.

I would like to thank the editors of my book, Drs. Steven M. Podos and Myron Yanoff, as well as Dr. George Bohegian, who made many useful suggestions. I would also like to acknowledge the help of Leah Kennedy, editorial director at Mosby-Year Book Europe, Ltd.

CONTENTS

1

Ethics in medicine is not a new topic. The Code of Hammurabi, a complex document written around 2,000 b.c. in Babylonia, is the first document that specifies in detail the conduct expected of a physician. The best known code of conduct, the Oath of Hippocrates, was developed in ancient Greece in the fifth century b.c. and, with minor revisions, has remained the expression of the ideals of ethical conduct for physicians today. It defines the essence of the caring physician, emphasizing that protection of patient rights is primary and that trustworthiness is an integral part of ethical conduct by a professional. When the American Medical Association was founded in 1847, it considered the establishment of a Code of Ethics one of its primary responsibilities. This code, based on the earlier writings of the English physician Thomas Percival, has remained the backbone of the current Principles of Medical Ethics used by the AMA today (Fig. 1.1).[1]

The American Academy of Ophthalmology has developed a Code of Ethics for its members, which is divided into two parts: Principles of Ethics, ideals to which all members *should* aspire (Fig. 1.2), and Rules of Ethics, an enforceable set of minimal standards to which all members *must* conform. The topics addressed include competence, informed consent, impaired ophthalmologists, preoperative assessment and postoperative care, and delegation of services. A complex system of administrative procedures has been developed to implement the Rules of Ethics, the primary emphasis being on modification of improper behavior rather than punitive action.[2]

Unethical conduct can be defined as actions that fail to conform to the standards, policies, procedures, and customs of a profession. It is important to realize that the ethical code for any profession may go beyond the laws, rules, and regulations of the states and federal government, but may not be in conflict with or less stringent than those regulations. If it is determined that such an ethical code does conflict with these rules, it is up to the courts and other government agencies to resolve the problem, their primary goal being protection of the "public good." Unfortunately, when government intervention occurs, the decision reached often protects neither the interests of the public nor those of the profession.

The primary difficulty encountered with both the AMA and AAO codes is not with their content but with their enforcement. The AMA and the AAO have no legal authority to suspend the right of an ophthalmologist to practice medicine. The only weapons available to modify behavior are peer pressure and, ultimately, expulsion from the organization. The former is often ineffective, and the latter not much of a penalty, since membership in the organizations is not necessary to retain licensure.

In addition, medical organizations have the obligation to report to appropriate government agencies "credible evidence" of criminal conduct on the part of a physician engaged in the practice of medicine. Conversely, the exoneration of a member physician in either civil or criminal judicial proceedings does not relieve or release the responsible professional organization

---

Figure 1.1. American Medical Association Principles of Medical Ethics

Preamble: The medical profession has long subscribed to a body of ethical statements developed primarily for the benefit of the patient. As a member of this profession, a physician must recognize responsibility not only to patients but also to society, to other health professionals, and to self. The following principles adopted by the American Medical Association are not laws, but standards of conduct which define the essentials of honorable behavior for the physician.

1. A physician shall be dedicated to providing competent medical service with compassion and respect for human dignity.

2. A physician shall deal honestly with patients and colleagues, and strive to expose those physicians deficient in character or competence, or who engage in fraud or deception.

3. A physician shall respect the law and also recognize a responsibility to seek changes in those requirements which are contrary to the best interests of the patient.

4. A physician shall respect the right of patients, of colleagues, and of other health professionals, and shall safeguard patient confidences within the constraints of the law.

5. A physician shall continue to study, apply, and advance scientific knowledge, make relevant information available to patients, colleagues, and the public, obtain consultation, and use the talents of other health professionals when indicated.

6. A physician shall, in the provision of appropriate patient care, except in emergencies, be free to choose whom to serve, with whom to associate, and the environment in which to provide medical services.

7. A physician shall recognize a responsibility to participate in the activities contributing to an improved community.

Reproduced by permission from the American Medical Association.

from disciplining that member if the actions in question violate ethical or professional standards.[1]

A national organization must also ensure that its Code of Ethics has the primary function of protecting the interests of the consumer rather than the profession and that it is not inherently anticompetitive in nature. To ensure that its code met these federally mandated criteria, the AAO submitted its Code of Ethics to the Federal Trade Commission for review. Subsequently, in 1983 the FTC issued an advisory opinion that the Code of Ethics of the Academy was not on its face anticompetitive,[2] and could be enforced on its members.

The Rules of Ethics of the American Academy of Ophthalmology deserve careful examination because they thoughtfully describe the conduct incumbent on the ethical ophthalmologist. The Rules of Conduct are summarized below, with direct quotes so indicated.

Copies of the Code of Ethics, which includes the administrative procedures to be followed for the enforcement of the Code, as well as the Practical Guide, which includes a series of advisory opinions and policy statements,

RULES OF ETHICS

Figure 1.2. Principles of Ethics of the American Academy of Ophthalmology

1. Ethics in Ophthalmology. Ethics are moral values. An issue of ethics in ophthalmology is resolved by the determination that the best interest of the patient is served.

2. Providing Ophthalmological Services. Ophthalmological services must be provided with compassion, respect for human dignity, honesty, and integrity.

3. Competence of the Ophthalmologist. An ophthalmologist must maintain competence by continued study. That competence must be supplemented with the talents of other professionals and with consultation when indicated.

4. Communication with the Patient. Open communication with the patient is essential. Patient confidences must be safeguarded within the constraints of the law.

5. Fees for Ophthalmological Services. Fees for ophthalmological services must not exploit patients or others who pay for the services.

6. Corrective Action. If a member has a reasonable basis for believing that another person has deviated from professionally accepted standards in a manner that adversely affects patient care or from the Rules of Ethics, the member should attempt to prevent the continuation of this conduct by communicating with the other person and/or identifying that person to the appropriate authorities and cooperating with those authorities in their professional and legal efforts to prevent the continuation of the conduct.

7. An Ophthalmologist's Responsibility. It is the responsibility of an ophthalmologist to act in the best interest of the patient.

Reproduced by permission from the American Academy of Ophthalmol-

are available from the American Academy of Ophthalmology, Membership Services Department, 655 Beach Street, San Francisco, CA 94120.

In the area of competence, it is stated that the ophthalmologist should perform only procedures for which his or her training and experience are sufficient and should not misrepresent "credentials, training, experience, ability or results." *Informed consent* must be obtained before the performance of all medical or surgical procedures. Along the same lines, *clinical experiments and investigative procedures* require approval via formal review mechanisms, with special attention to informed consent under these special circumstances.

Proper *preoperative assessment* requires adequate evaluation of the physical condition of patients, as well as their social, emotional, and occupational needs. "Performance of unnecessary surgery is an extremely serious ethical violation." The operating surgeon must adequately and accurately document the indications for surgery.

The provision of *postoperative care* remains the responsibility of the operating surgeon until such time as the patient is sufficiently recovered, and the operating surgeon must provide all aspects of care that are within the unique competence of the ophthalmologist. In an emergency, alternate arrangements can be made as long as the welfare of the patient is the primary consideration. Fee arrangements between the operating surgeon and the provider of postoperative care should be revealed to the patient in advance. It is permissible for the ophthalmologist to be involved in *delegation of services* to others, as long as the individuals to whom those services are delegated are both qualified and adequately supervised. In the event of an emergency, proper treatment and the welfare of the patient should be the only considerations in deciding to whom the care will be entrusted.

An ophthalmologist must not *misrepresent* the medical or surgical procedure that is being performed, who will be performing the procedure, or the charges that will be incurred for the service(s) rendered. In addition, no ophthalmologist should benefit from a *commercial relationship* at the expense of the patient's welfare and rights, and only *procedures and materials* that are required for proper treatment of the patient should be used.

Communications to colleagues should be both accurate and truthful, and *communications to the public* must not "convey false, untrue, deceptive or misleading information through statements, testimonials, photographs, graphics or other means." They should not create the impression that results can be guaranteed, and must explain, in addition to the benefits of a procedure, the alternatives and significant risks associated with it. They must accurately describe the training and experience of the ophthalmologist, and "must not contain material claims of superiority that cannot be substantiated."

Disclosures of professionally related commercial interests to all relevant parties (including patients, colleagues, and the public) are required, and all *interrelationships among ophthalmologists* should be governed with the best interests of the patient in mind.

The *impaired ophthalmologist* (physically, mentally, or emotionally) should refrain from practicing ophthalmology until the impairment no longer compromises patient welfare. Any ophthalmologist who is aware of a practicing but impaired ophthalmologist is ethically bound to take whatever action is necessary to ensure his or her withdrawal from practice.

The difficulty in enforcing a code of ethics becomes even more apparent as medicine shifts (or perhaps is being shifted) from a profession to a business, since business ethics and professional ethics are distinctly different and in many instances contradictory. As defined by Webster's Dictionary, a profession is a "calling requiring specialized knowledge and often long and extensive academic training." A business, in contrast, is defined in the same source as a "commercial or mercantile activity engaged in as a means of livelihood."

In the past, the necessity of making such a distinction was not essential because the concept of the practice of medicine as a learned profession was taken for granted. As a result, regulation of professional activities was usually left in the hands of the profession itself. It was felt that the standards set by self regulation of the profession would be in general higher than those imposed on commercial conduct, and that those most familiar with the field (i.e., the professionals) would best understand the nuances that contribute to a responsible code of conduct. Furthermore, it was assumed that members of a "learned profession," unlike those involved in pure commercial activity, could be trusted to suppress self interest in favor of the patient.

The separation of the practice of medicine from the commercial aspects of payment for medical services has never been complete or even clear-cut. The dual themes relating professions to knowledge and dedicated service on the one hand, and trading of technical skills and advice for payment on the other, have always placed professions midway between a pure "calling" and a trade.[3]

Recent changes in both the legal and medical fields have further blurred the distinction between medicine as a profession and medicine as a trade, creating problems for patients, physicians, and entities such as insurance carriers and regulatory agencies that are at the interface between the two. These changes include: the development of alternative health care financing systems that intrude on and often disrupt the traditional doctor–patient relationship; large nationwide hospital chains (often for-profit); aggressive advertising by outpatient surgical and treatment centers; and the tendency of the public to regard medical care as a commodity to be shopped for rather than a professional service to be delivered.

Additional changes more specific to ophthalmology have been: the refinement of cataract surgery techniques and skills to the point that the procedure can be safely performed in an outpatient setting, with prompt rehabilitation of the patient; development of networks between certain ophthalmologists and other providers who agree to refer patients in return for other considerations; refinement and active promotion of refractive surgical techniques as an alternative to glasses or contact lenses on otherwise healthy eyes; and the general tendency of many ophthalmologists to consider cataract surgery as the "be all and end all" of ophthalmologic practice. This latter trend (which may be encouraged by training programs with very few general ophthalmologists to serve as role models), coupled with an increasing tendency for many high-volume cataract surgeons to advertise and promote their practices aggressively, has significantly altered the doctor–patient relationship. Longstanding associations between physicians and patients disappear as a result of these influences.

It is fair to say that not all of the changes described have been detrimental to the patient or the ophthalmologist; however, they have significantly altered the practice of ophthalmology. Some of the more important trends and their causes are discussed below.

THE BUSINESS OF MEDICINE

ANTITRUST CONSIDERATIONS

For many years the professions were held to be exempt from the provisions of the Sherman Antitrust Act (1890) and the Clayton Act (1914). The key provisions of these acts outlawed contracts and conspiracies, tie-in arrangements, and monopolistic practices that restrained trade and competition. There was little application of these laws to medicine for many years because it was felt that the relationship between patient and physician was different from that encountered in most commercial matters.[4] Anticompetitive activities such as licensure, specialty certification, and accreditation of training programs were believed to preserve adequate professional standards, thus protecting the public without primarily benefiting the practitioners.[3] The exemption was allowed despite the fact that *all* professions are by their nature inherently monopolistic because they restrict both supply and external competition, limit access, and may actually raise costs above those that would exist in a truly competitive market.

The practice of considering professions as trades, and thus subject to antitrust considerations, started in earnest in 1975, when the Supreme Court ruled that professions such as medicine and law were not exempt from the Sherman Antitrust Act (Goldfarb v. Virginia State Bar). This opinion, which indicated that lawyers in Virginia were liable for price-fixing charges in title search activities, meant that all professions were subject to challenge under the antitrust laws if their code of ethics or other rules and regulations were thought to stifle competition.

This decision and the others that followed established the basis on which all professions are evaluated—that all rules and regulations of a given profession, no matter what their source or intended purpose, must actually serve to assist the profession in its primary function: service of the public good. Any rule that fails to do so and instead diminishes competition among individual practitioners usually will not survive a legal challenge (e.g., Boddicker v. Arizona Dental Association).[2]

THE FEDERAL TRADE COMMISSION

The Federal Trade Commission (FTC) is the agency in charge of regulating activities under the various antitrust acts. After the Supreme Court rulings discussed above, the FTC soon decreed that physician advertising could not be prohibited as a matter of course and that ethical codes limiting advertising by physicians were anticompetitive unless they were demonstrably necessary to protect patients. In 1982 the Supreme Court let stand a lower court decision finding the AMA in restraint of trade because its code of ethics strictly prohibited physician advertising and the solicitation of patients. This decision also provided that patient solicitation and arrangements between physicians and nonphysicians which were not harmful in any way to consumers could not be prohibited as a matter of course and that ethical guidelines pertaining to this area must first be approved by the FTC (FTC v. AMA 1982).

These policies were developed in the hope that advertising and various other referral arrangements would encourage competition and drive down the cost of medical care by subjecting it to the same market forces as any other commodity. It was believed that if advertising were allowed patients could shop for price and thus decrease medical costs. As discussed earlier, however, it is clear (in hindsight, at least) that the transformation of medicine from its traditional mode of practice to its formal recognition as a business created increased demand for services without a corresponding decrease in cost and also produced the host of other problems with which we are struggling today.

The system that currently exists is the framework within which all of us must work. With that in mind, it is important to discuss some of the ethical considerations that must be regarded as an integral part of the practice of medicine, regardless of whether it is considered a profession, a business, or a hybrid. These guidelines, provided to help define what constitutes "ethical practice," are highly subjective in many instances, and "ethical practitioners" may disagree quite strongly on specific points. Therefore, although the material that follows primarily represents the author's personal opinion, it is hoped that it also represents the viewpoint of the majority of "mainstream" ophthalmologists.

Many ethical considerations are obvious. The interests of the patient must be paramount and protected at all cost. All tests and procedures must be performed with the welfare of the patient in mind, without regard for financial reward to the physician or similar considerations. Patient confidentiality must also be protected. The use of testimonials and/or the listing of patients as references (if necessary at all) must be done only with the written permission of the patient. Several other specific considerations are discussed in greater detail below.

GUIDELINES FOR ETHICAL BEHAVIOR

MARKETING AND ADVERTISING

Advertising and marketing programs should primarily provide information for patients and should not represent the physician as having unique skills and abilities or as being superior to other similarly trained and credentialed physicians. The ads should also not guarantee results or represent medical procedures as painless, risk-free, or simple. The American Society of Cataract and Refractive Surgeons has developed voluntary guidelines for advertising cataract and refractive surgery which are quite useful.[5] Without taking a position on whether members should actually advertise, they describe principles that are consistent with AAO ethical standards and yet allow active and efficient use of various promotional materials. *The Guide*,[6] a publication of the AAO, also has a module on marketing that describes many ethical and effective marketing tools.

Most importantly, advertising materials should not induce a patient to agree to a medically unnecessary procedure. This concept is one of the most important differences between an ethical medical advertisement and one employed in simple commerce. It is not the job of a salesperson to evaluate the customer's need for a given service or product (have you ever heard a car salesman tell you that the old one is fine and you should come back in a year or two?). A salesperson is not expected to be impartial or to give automatically a good, fair deal; he has a significant financial interest in the outcome. It is the consumer's responsibility to appraise each situation, compare offers, and make a suitable choice.

The situation in medicine is quite different. Here the physician (with only the best interests of the patient in mind) must both help to determine whether or not a service is necessary and then assist the patient (who is not a customer!) in reaching the best decision. We have all had patients say, "I'll do whatever you tell me, doctor." The trust inherent in that statement cannot be betrayed.

The primary beneficiary in the doctor–patient interaction must be the patient—not the physician, the physician's employees, or vendors of ophthalmic products. *Caveat emptor*, although recognized as a business truism, has no place in the practice of medicine. The patient should never have to wonder if the physician has an ulterior motive in suggesting a specific treatment plan. Offering employees bonuses for "rounding up" patients for elective procedures or exerting undue pressure on patients to make particular decisions is unethical and deplorable.

Although advertising and marketing are approved practices, they may not be medically beneficial. Commercial advertising may help patients by making them aware of various available options, but it runs the risk of delivering incomplete and misleading information. The intent of commercial advertising, in fact, is often deliberately deceptive, because "telling the truth" may discourage use of the advertised product. Although the average consumer understands that a significant amount of hyperbole exists in pure commercial advertising, medical advertising may not be assessed as skeptically. The degree to which physicians are respected as ethical practitioners may lead patients to assume that the information contained in their promotional materials is complete and accurate.

The promotion of services should be distinguished from advertising of products such as glasses, contact lenses, and other appliances for which a consumer can make a reasonably enlightened evaluation of need and comparison among alternative sources of supply.

Advertising and marketing by physicians also is different from commercial advertising because patients are purchasing a service for which someone else is usually paying most of the cost. Therefore, an unneeded or marginally necessary service will likely be purchased if it is presented attractively. Patients who take little personal financial risk probably will be less inclined to evaluate critically the purchase of a service than persons paying their own bills.[7] When a procedure is presented as "safe, painless, risk-free" *and free*, demand for it is very likely to increase.

The situation is further complicated by the fact that the "supply" of cataracts is essentially endless in the elderly population and there is no shortage of ophthalmologists available to remove them. If supply is not fixed and demand increases for any reason (including advertising and/or marketing), overall costs associated with removal of these cataracts will probably increase, even if the payment for each cataract removed decreases. Under these circumstances, the competition envisioned by the FTC when it encouraged physician advertising has not resulted in decreased costs.

In addition to advertising, various marketing techniques for patients, such as vans for transportation, have been developed. These should be offered for the genuine convenience of the patients and not to keep them from stopping somewhere else to receive care. Referral arrangements with nonmedical providers involving delegation of postoperative care to someone of lesser training and experience should be done only with the best interest of the patient in mind and not to enhance the relationship with the referral source to encourage the supply of additional patients. Financial incentives granted to referral sources to develop or maintain that relationship are unethical and often illegal.

HIGH-VOLUME SURGEONS

The volume of surgery performed is not, in and of itself, the primary issue, but the appropriateness of the surgery and level of care provided before, during, and after surgery are of paramount importance. This was emphasized by an AAO representative in his testimony before the Subcommittee on Health, House Ways and Means Committee in June 1990, who stated, "Volume in itself is not necessarily a bad thing. But, we are strongly opposed to selling cataract surgery like a commodity, and to engaging in a volume of service so high that the surgeon cannot personally provide complete care."[8]

At the same hearing, a representative of the Inspector General's office dealt with the subject of Medicare fraud, waste, and abuse among high-volume providers (defined as ophthalmologists or groups of ophthalmologists receiving over $1 million from Medicare in 1987). High-volume surgery, he stated, was twice as likely not to meet minimal clinical thresholds for necessity; twice as likely to be of poor quality; more likely to be of questionable quality; less likely to have intraoperative complications; more likely to have postoperative complications; twice as likely to be performed on patients with visual acuity of 20/40 or better; and less likely to result in improved visual acuity.[9]

There is no evidence, however, that an independent review of the same data would come to an identical conclusion. A recent analysis of the information contained in the report suggests that several of the opinions expressed were incorrect.[10] Nevertheless, the association of high operative volume with poor quality of and questionable indications for surgery mentioned in the report raises the possibility that, in some instances, less than optimal care could occur because of the volume of cases performed. That the charge was raised at all should remind every ophthalmologist to take sufficient time preoperatively and personally determine that:

1. The patient has decreased acuity that interferes with functional ability, occupation, lifestyle, or important activities
2. A cataract is present that is dense enough to account for all or most of the visual impairment
3. Removal of the cataract is likely to result in improved functional visual capacity
4. Proper informed consent regarding the realistic benefits and possible complications of the procedure has been obtained

It is also proper to remove cataracts that interfere with the diagnosis and/or treatment of additional ocular disease, or which are themselves causing problems (as in phacoanaphylaxis) even if visual improvement will not occur.

There is a danger in the recent trend, which has been spurred on by the rules and regulations of the federal government, to separate the technical aspects of cataract removal from the practice of medicine as a profession. Preoperative evaluation and postoperative care may now be legally (if not properly) delegated to nonphysicians. Eye care networks have been developed that provide patients to certain chosen ophthalmic surgeons, and patients may be operated on and never seen again by the operating surgeon except under unusual circumstances.

It is not going to take long for someone (read this as the government and other third-party payors) to figure out that maybe you don't have to be a physician at all to remove cataracts if primarily technical—not medical—skills are involved. Perhaps a surgical technician could be trained to perform the same procedure at a much lower price, with referral to ophthalmologists only if problems develop. Salaried nonmedical personnel could be employed for preoperative evaluation to avoid potential economic conflict of interest and could deliver routine postoperative care, with referral to ophthalmologists for complications. Ophthalmologists could easily be left out of the loop entirely and have no one but some of our brethren to blame.

THE COST OF HEALTH CARE

The socioeconomic aspects of medical care in the United States are assuming an increasingly important place in the practice of medicine. This is due primarily to the rapid and seemingly endless increase in health care costs despite vigorous efforts to contain them. In 1970 total national health care expenditures were approximately $70 billion. In 1992 the costs exceeded $800 billion, and are expected to top $900 billion in 1993.[1] This increase, an average annual rate of 17%, exceeds the rate of growth of the consumer price index (CPI) by a factor of 2.[2] In terms of the gross domestic product (GDP), the change is from 7.4% of GDP to 14% in 1992 (Fig. 2.1). Therefore, the rate of increase in health care spending is greater than the rate of growth of the GDP (Fig. 2.2), indicating to some that health care expenses are consuming an increasing share of the nation's economic resources and are one of the major reasons for the large federal budget deficit in recent years. Because of this, President Clinton pledged to make health care reform one of his primary objectives during the first 100 days of his presidency, and his wife Hillary Rodham Clinton heads the task force to guide the way.[3]

Analysis of data derived from the National Medical Expenditure Survey[4] indicates that 30% of the total dollars spent on health care in 1987 were used to provide services for the sickest 1% of the population. The top 5% accounted for almost 60% of the total. Almost half of those patients were over the age of 65, even though only 11% of the general population fall into that category. The bottom 50% of the population consumed less than 5% of all medical resources.

Information developed by the AMA Center for Health Policy Research[1] also provides useful material about the breakdown in spending for medical care. It confirms that a relatively small proportion of individuals with severe health problems consume most of the nation's health care dollars. In those under the age of 65, 10% of the population accounts for 75% of the expense; in those over age 65, 25% of the population accounts for 90% of all medical expenditures. Hospital costs account for 40% of total payments and physician costs 20%. Even more striking is the fact that 4% of Medicare beneficiaries account for 50% of total Medicare payments, and the 6% who die each year account for about 25% of Medicare expenses during their last year of life.

This study also documents how significantly health care costs increase with age. Medicare beneficiaries constitute about 12% of the population but generate 36% of all personal health care expenses. Per capita costs for those

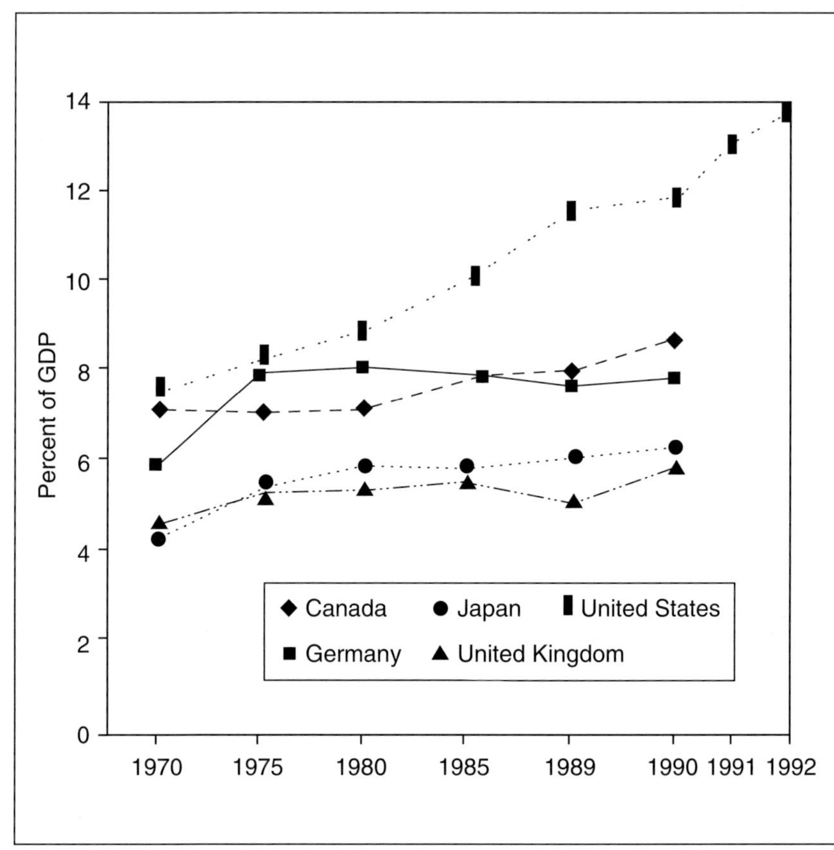

2.1 | Health expenditures as a percentage of gross domestic product, for U.S. and selected countries, 1980–1992. (*Note:* Gross domestic product (GDP) is equal to gross national product less net property income from abroad. *Source:* Scheiber and Poullier 1991; Organization for Economic Cooperation and Development, Health Data File, 1991. Adapted from Physician Payment Review Commission, Annual Report, 1993, p. 2.)

under age 65 are $1,268; the per capita costs for those over age 65 are $5,360, three times the national average. For those over age 85 the outlay increases to 750% of the national average, with 40% of the total representing nursing

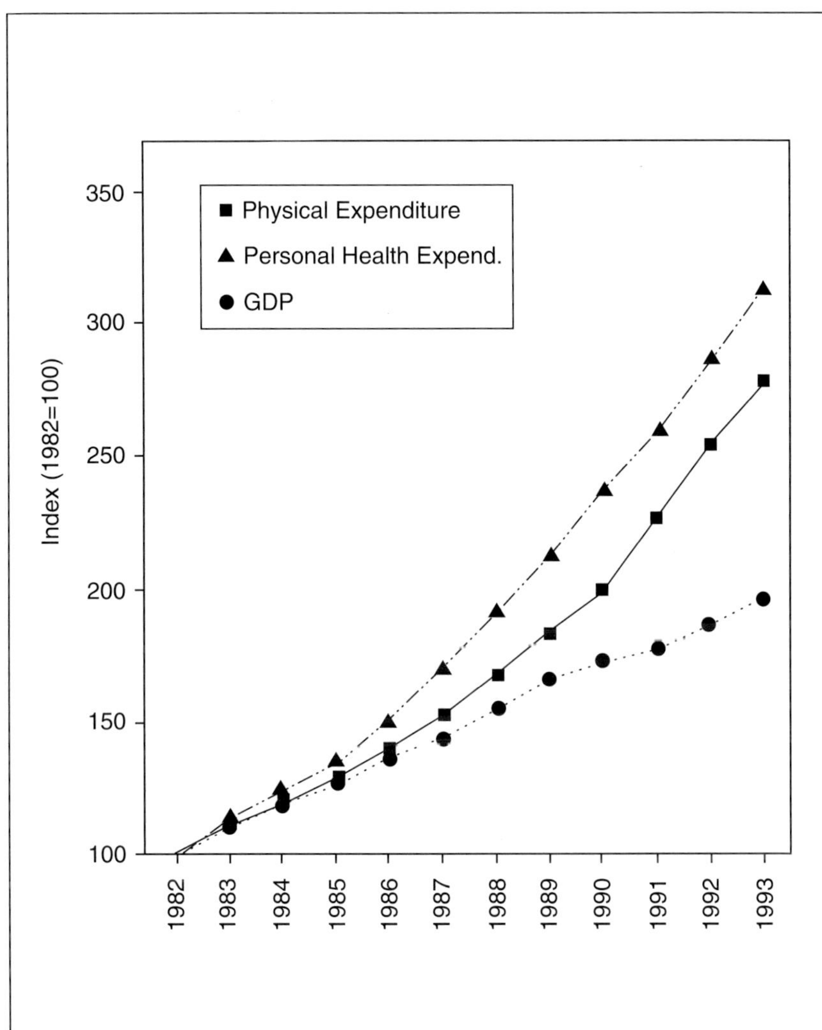

2.2 | Trends in physician expenditures, personal health expenditures, and gross domestic product, 1982–1993. (*Note:* Data for 1992 and 1993 are projected. *Source:* Congressional Budget Office. Adapted from PPRC Report to Congress, 1993, p. 3.)

home expenses. Some of the other factors that account for the growth of health care spending are outlined in Figure 2.3.

In 1992, total health care expenditures per capita for those of all ages rose to $3,160, an increase of 11.5% from 1991. The estimated health care bill for the average family was $4,260, which included taxes related to medical care (39%), out-of-pocket costs (32%), insurance premiums (17%), and Medicare taxes and premiums (12%).[5]

Costs for physician services continue to increase at a rate higher than the Consumer Price Index (CPI); however, the rate of increase is moderating. In 1992, these costs increased by 6.3%, less than the average of 7.4% during the 1980s (Fig. 2.4). Some of this moderation is due to the increasing control over payments by third-party payers, regardless of actual increase in charges. As noted by one physician, "Health care is becoming like so many industries, where no one pays the list price." The lower inflation rate, increased number of salaried physicians, and improved productivity and cost efficiency have also had a favorable impact.[6]

The growth of the portion of the GDP related to medical expenses does have a bright side. The health care industry has become a leading contributor to the economy. It is predicted that health care spending will account for 25% to 33% of the growth of the GDP over the next 5 years.[7] In 1988, 7 million individuals worked at jobs related to health care. At present, 10 million Americans work in hospitals, pharmacies, nursing homes, and other health-related areas, an annual growth rate of 9.3%.[5] In many cities, including Detroit, Cleveland, and St. Louis, the health care industry is the major employer. The industry is labor intensive and provides good jobs with excellent fringe benefits for many minorities. Reductions in health care spending will necessarily result in a loss of many of these jobs, which will not be easy to replace in the current economic climate.[8]

Provision of eye care comprises a major portion of the health care industry. The optical market in 1991, which includes dispensing and sale of frames, prescription spectacle lenses, and contact lenses, was over $12 billion. The purchase of nonprescription sunglasses ($1.75 billion) and over-the-counter reading glasses ($200 million), as well as the provision of eye examinations ($3.5 billion), brought the total ophthalmic market to almost $16 billion.[9] When the surgical and medical treatment of eye disease is added, the total exceeds $20 billion.

FIGURE 2.3. Factors Accounting for Growth in Health Care Spending, 1985–1990

Service	Population Increase	General Inflation	Medical Price Inflation	Utilization of Services	Intensity of Services	Total
Inpatient	+12.7%	+44.6%	+24.5%	−23.2%	41.4%	100%
Outpatient	+6.0%	+21.2%	+11.6%	+30.6%	30.6%	100%
Physicians	+8.3%	+29.2%	+21.4%	+3.7%	37.4%	100%
Nursing homes	+10.9%	+38.4%	+15.4%	+2.6%	32.7%	100%

Source: U.S. Industrial Outlook—1993, Health and Medical Services, p. 42.2.

The Medicare program was developed in 1965 to assist elderly Americans with the payment of medical expenses. Its rapid growth, from $35 billion in 1980 (6% of the federal budget) to $131 billion in 1992 (8%), has made it the fastest growing component of the federal budget. The program, divided into parts A and B, is funded through a combination of payroll taxes, beneficiary premiums, and general revenue. At present there are approximately 34 million enrollees. These include persons aged 65 and above, disabled individuals, and most of those with end-stage kidney disease.[5] A summary of the benefits is shown in Figure 2.5.

PAYMENT OF HEALTH CARE EXPENSES
FEDERAL GOVERNMENT EXPENSES

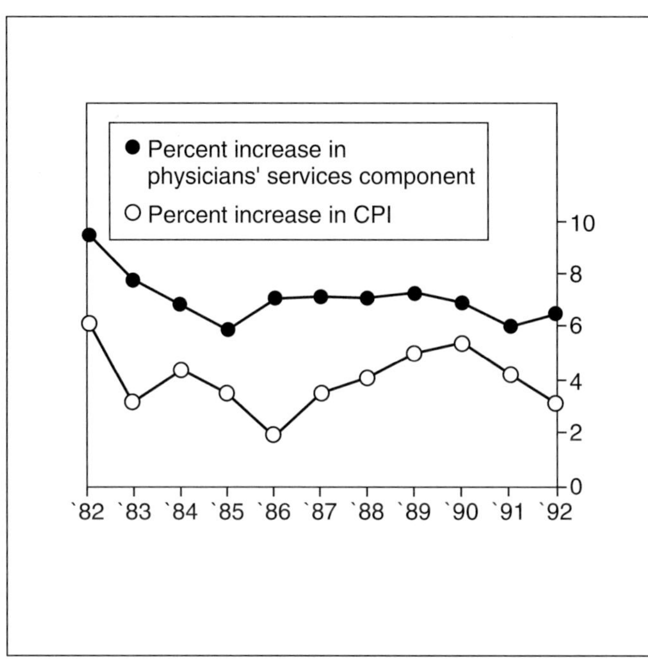

2.4 | Slowdown in growth in cost of physician services. (*Source:* U.S. Department of Labor, Bureau of Labor Statistics, Washington D.C. From *American Medical News,* Feb 8, 1993, p. 16.)

FIGURE 2.5. Cost Sharing Under Medicare, 1993

	BENEFICIARY LIABILITY
Medicare, Part A	
Hospital deductible	$676 per spell of illness
Hospital coinsurance	
Days 61–90	$169 per day
Days 90 on (for 60 lifetime reserve days)	$338 per day
Skilled nursing facility coinsurance Days 21–100	$84.50 per day
Medicare, Part B	
Premium	$36.60 per month
Deductible	$100 per year
Coinsurance	20% of allowed charge
Balance bills	All excess up to 115% allowed charge for nonparticipating physicians

Adapted from PPRC, Report to Congress, 1992.

Part A [officially called hospital insurance (HI)] covers payments for care provided by hospitals, skilled nursing facilities, home health agencies, and hospice programs. It is funded largely by a 1.45% Social Security payroll tax levied on both employees and employers. At present the wage base for this tax is just over $135,000, but removal of this limit has been proposed for the future. Part A expenditures in 1992 totaled $82.9 billion, an increase of $11.3 billion over 1991 (+15.8%). Most of the increase was due to the rapid growth of utilization of skilled nursing facilities and home health programs.[10]

Part B [Supplementary Medical Insurance (SMI)] covers physicians' services, laboratory fees, outpatient hospital services, end-stage renal disease, and durable medical equipment. It is paid for by a combination of general revenues (73%), enrollee premiums (23%), and interest payments paid to the Medicare Trust Fund (3%).[11] The monthly premium for 1993 is $36.60, and patients also pay an annual $100 deductible.

In 1992 the spending for Part B was $49.2 billion, an increase of only 5.3% over 1991. This was the lowest annual increase in more than a decade. The implementation of the Resource Based Relative Value Scale (RBRVS), discussed in greater detail later, undoubtedly played a significant role in reducing the rate of increase. The volume of physicians' services also increased less than predicted, which also helped to contain costs.

Payments to ophthalmologists constitute a significant portion of overall part B payments to physicians. Between 1983 and 1986 the number of cataract procedures performed per 1,000 Medicare beneficiaries increased by almost 50%. The change in case mix during the same period (the substitution of cataract extraction with lens implant for extraction only) increased actual expenditures by 61%. During the same period, the actual allowed charges per beneficiary increased by 57.3% (twice the rate for all physicians), with the excess due almost entirely to cataract surgery.[12]

Data provided by the federal Health Care Finance Administration (HCFA) indicate that 1,322,979 cataract extractions with lens implant (CPT 66984) were billed to Medicare in 1989. In 1990, "only" 1,063,431 were performed. Despite the decrease, the procedure remained the number one Medicare surgical procedure, with allowed charges of $1.66 billion dollars. Yag capsulotomy (CPT 66821) was number two (512,104, or $300 million). These procedures together accounted for over 22% of the payments to *all* surgeons in 1990. Panretinal photocoagulation ranked ninth, and laser trabeculoplasty was tenth (114,771, or $103 million), accounting for just over 2.5%. Yag capsulotomies, however, increased by 53% between 1988 and 1990, and laser trabeculoplasties increased by 29%. Only 12,000 intracapsular cataract extractions were performed.

Payments for medical eye services also represented a significant expense for Medicare. More than 6 million comprehensive eye exams were performed in 1990.[13] Between 1986 and 1989 the annualized growth rate for medical eye services was 18%, higher than any other group of services studied.[14] These trends help to explain why ophthalmology has been targeted by HCFA in recent years when cost control mechanisms are instituted. As an example, several years ago cataract surgery, along with 26 other ophthalmologic procedures, was placed on the list of "overpriced procedures" subject to special fee reductions (10% or more for cataract surgery). Subsequent implementation of the RBRVS then decreased the fees even more.

The federal government also has health care responsibilities outside of the Medicare program. Medicaid is a federally supported, state-administered program that provides medical care for low-income individuals, persons receiving Aid to Families with Dependent Children, and disabled individuals. At present the Medicaid program is responsible for over 16% of personal health care spending in the United States. The f ederal government pays more than half of the cost, which in 1992 totaled $114 billion for approximately 28 million eligible individuals. Only 6% of that total was paid to physicians. It is estimated that the overall cost for 1993 will be close to $140 billion and that Medicaid costs will soon exceed those for Medicare if present trends continue.

The elderly consume an inordinate share of the Medicaid budget, with expenses in 1991 for the older individuals averaging $8,524, in contrast to $1,086 for children and $1,844 for younger adults in low-income families. Eligibility rules and application procedures are complicated, which probably prevents many people who qualify for benefits from enrolling. Income for eligibility varies from state to state, as do benefits per capita, which ranged from a high of $5,994 in Connecticut to a low of $1,607 in Mississippi. Only half of Americans with incomes below the federal poverty level are actually eligible for benefits.[15]

Medicaid expenditures increased $37 billion between 1988 and 1991. The reasons for this include increased numbers of eligible persons because of expansion of the program to include all low-income pregnant women, inclusion of Medicare premiums for certain elderly patients, and the recession with its accompanying high level of unemployment (causing loss of health insurance in addition to wages). Medicaid is also the primary payer for long-term nursing home care for those who have no other means available, for home health care, and for intermediate care facility costs for the mentally retarded. These three areas account for over 41% of total disbursements.

Rising Medicaid expenditures also have an impact on state budgets. This is due in part to the federal legislative mandates discussed above, which have increased the number of eligible beneficiaries, expanded benefits, and increased administrative burdens without a commensurate increase in federal funding.[16] In Missouri, for example, the state portion of the Medicaid payment will rise $213 million starting in fiscal 1994 (July 1993). This increase will bring the state contribution to $477 million and make Medicaid the second largest expenditure in the state's $10 billion budget.[17] This experience is not unique to Missouri. With expenses rising at an annual rate of 15%, many states will be forced to cut other services or raise taxes to keep pace with their health care costs. For this reason, state governors have joined forces to urge the federal government to increase federal contributions to the Medicaid program and to push rapidly for additional programs for health care reform.

MEDICAID (FEDERAL AND STATE)

PRIVATE INDUSTRY AND LABOR
INDUSTRY

The federal and state governments are not the only institutions that face rising health care expenses. Costs for private industry are also skyrocketing. As shown in Figure 2.6, annual health plan expenses per employee have continued to rise, reaching $4,000 in 1992. This represents an increase of almost $400 compared with 1991. The rate of increase has slowed to 12% to 13% after annual rises in previous years of close to 20%. The expense in 1993 is likely to approach $4,400.[18] Employers attempting to limit exposure are turning to cost-saving techniques such as increasing deductibles, co-payments, and out-of-pocket limits, and are asking employees to contribute a portion of the premium for themselves and/or their dependents.[19]

American manufacturers, such as the auto industry, claim that the increased medical costs they now face make them less competitive in the international marketplace. Health care costs add from $800 to $1,000 to the cost of each car manufactured in the United States.[20] In February of 1993, General Motors, which has a current annual health care expense of $3.4 billion for 1.8 million active and retired workers, took a charge against earnings for future health care costs of $22 billion for retirees alone.[21] Although this action had no tangible effect on the day-to-day operations of the company (which actually showed a small operating profit in the preceding quarter), its sheer magnitude caught the attention of Congress and other interested parties and will no doubt be used as additional ammunition in the push for future reform of the health care system.

Companies have adopted various strategies to deal with increasing health care costs. General Motors is attempting to cut the benefits for its non-union employees by requiring them for the first time to make a contribution for medical insurance coverage. It is also trying to limit benefits for

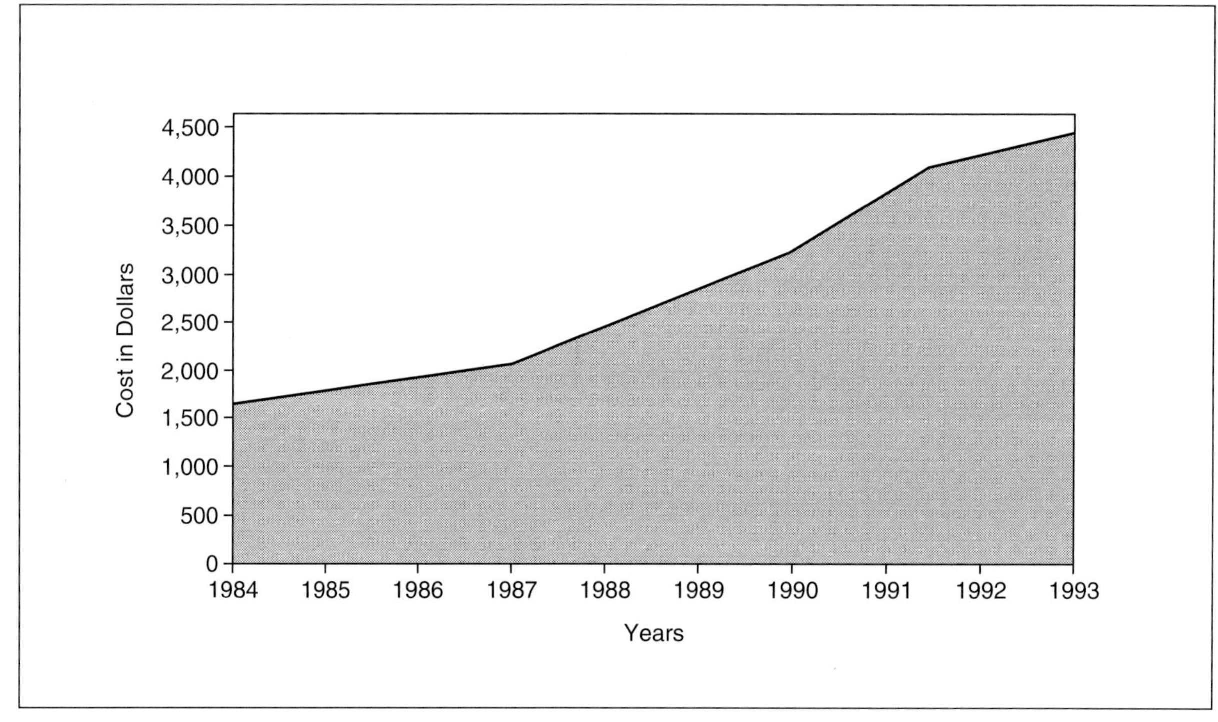

2.6 | Annual health plan cost per employee, 1984–1993. (*Source:* A. Foster Higgins & Co., Inc.)

retirees.[22] Other large companies (PepsiCo and Southwestern Bell, for example) have contracted with national networks of physicians and hospitals that provide favorable rates in return for receiving a significant portion of the health care concession.[23] Allied Signal has even developed a plan under which its insurance carrier agrees to absorb much of the cost if plan expenses rise above a predetermined level.

Xerox has also adopted an aggressive position with regard to controlling health care expenses. The company offers strong financial incentives for its employees to join Health Maintenence Organizations (HMOs) that have met strict standards for service and cost controls. The difference in premium for an individual who chooses a traditional insurance plan over the HMO option is almost $120 per month. Even though over two thirds of the employees have chosen the HMO option, expenses are still expected to increase by 12% in 1993.[24] Obviously, HMOs alone are not the answer.

Industry also pays a greater share of the health care dollar because of the payment policies of the federal government. Medicare pays only 90% of the true hospital costs for its enrollees, and Medicaid reimbursement is even lower (80%). Therefore, private payors must pick up the excess and are stuck with paying 128% of the cost, further increasing their expenses in an already overloaded situation.[26] They also pay higher fees for office visits and other outpatient procedures, because physicians have a fee schedule for private patients higher than that dictated by Medicare regulations.

The medical portion of Worker's Compensation Insurance has also become an increasing burden for the business community. Approximately 40% of the $40 billion spent yearly to compensate injured employees is spent on medical bills. The annual rate of increase in the medical portion of Workers' Compensation costs (11%) is even greater than that for general heath care costs (8%). To combat this trend, companies are beginning to spend more time and money on safety-related issues and risk management in an effort to decrease the chance of workplace-related injuries. They are also starting to place limits on physician fees and are demanding better documentation and justification for hospitalization and surgical treatment.[25]

Fraud and abuse are also rampant in many areas, with unscrupulous workers, attorneys, and physicians all involved in cheating the system. In some instances claimants have been told what their injuries were on the way to the physician's office, where they picked up claim forms that had already been filled out. In addition, as unemployment rises, the frequency of Workers' Compensation claims appears to be increasing. In California, one insurance carrier estimated that 40% of the claims filed involved plant closings, with up to 95% of the workers involved filing for benefits. The most common injury claims in this situation relate to stress and repetitive motion problems.[26]

LABOR

Labor unions, long successful in securing comprehensive health benefits for their members through collective bargaining agreements, are now also feeling the pinch. Obtaining and maintaining high-quality health insurance as a fringe benefit have been key considerations in many recent labor–management negotiations. Because of the importance of health care benefits to workers, lower wages and other concessions have been accepted in lieu of cuts in health care coverage or increases in cost sharing.[27]

Because of the tax-free nature of many fringe benefits, they comprise an increasing percentage of the total compensation package for both salaried and hourly workers. Department of Labor statistics indicate that, on average, over 27% of labor costs are in the form of benefits (Fig. 2.7). Unionized workers earn a higher percentage of compensation as benefits than non-union workers (33% versus 25%). Conversely, wage costs are, at a minimum, only 73% of the true cost of hiring an employee. Therefore, a wage of $13.00 per hour can translate into a true cost to the employer of almost $19.[28]

A recent article indicates that spending for health care for workers averages about about 7% of total labor costs. However, the recession has caused corporate profits to shrink, and because health care costs continue to rise rapidly they constitute a significant percentage of both pre- and post-tax profits (61.1% and 107.9%, respectively, in 1990).[29] Although many companies complain that this represents a significant drain on corporate resources and keeps them from being competitive, that argument is somewhat misleading since, overall, the contribution by business to employee benefits (including health care) constitutes only 1% of all corporate deductions to

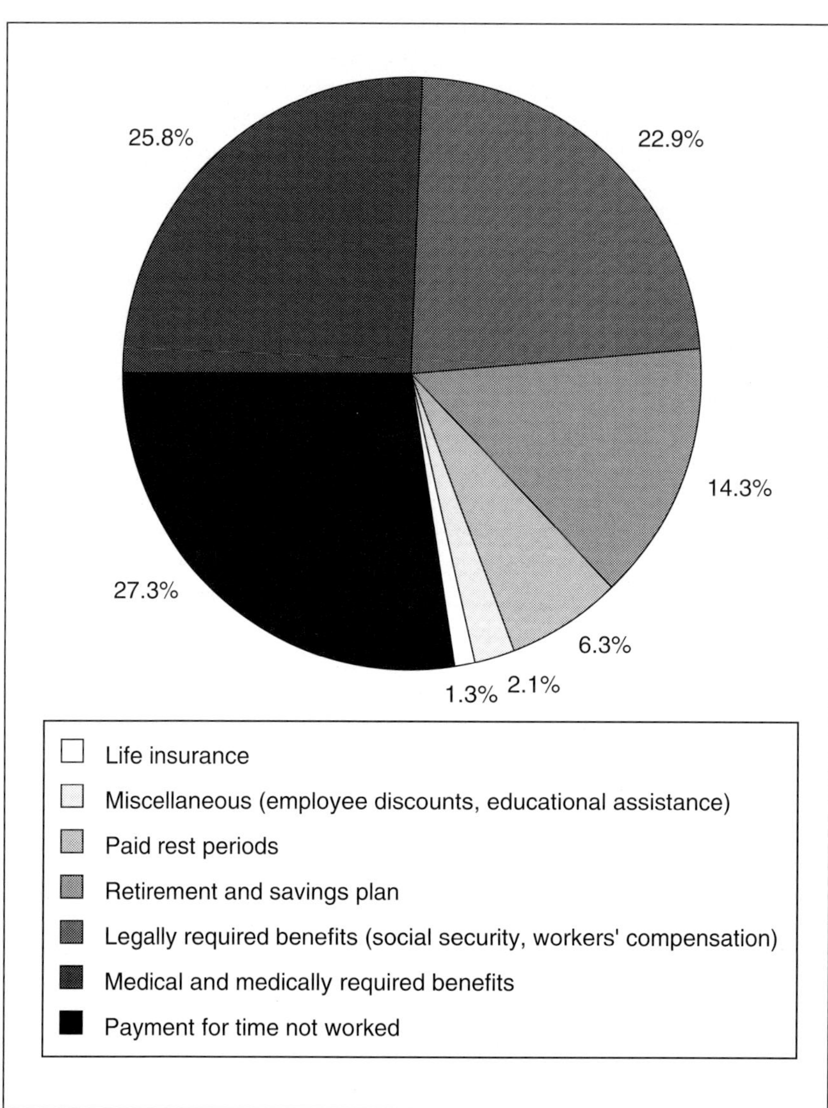

2.7 | Breakdown of the benefit dollar. (*Source:* U.S. Chamber of Commerce. From *Business and Health,* Mar 1992.)

income.[30] Since health benefits are only a portion of the overall compensation package for workers, it is probable that wages would be significantly higher if health care benefits were reduced, and therefore that the overall cost for workers would be little different from what it is now.

Not only active workers are affected. Many companies are beginning to ask retirees to pay a greater portion of their medical insurance premiums, and some companies, when they are legally allowed to, are eliminating benefits entirely. These workers constitute an easier target becuase current workers are often guaranteed benefits by contract. In addition, changes of benefits for active employees risk their alienation, thus creating a less productive work force. Many retirees are not taking these changes lightly, and litigation over preservation of benefits is becoming increasingly more common.[31]

The reasons for the increase in health care costs are multiple and complex. Such costs are driven upwards by consumers, physicians, manufacturers, home health and nursing home providers, and administrative costs inherent in the complex system under which we presently function. Several of the more important causes are discussed below.

It is clear that overutilization of some services by both physicians[32] and consumers can contribute to rising health care expenditures. In many cases there is no incentive for patients to control costs because they are insulated from them by first-dollar insurance coverage. A fee-for-service payment program also has the potential for physician abuse in an attempt to increase revenues. Several studies, for example, have shown that physicians who own imaging centers order more studies than those who do not.[33] No evidence was presented to indicate that the extra tests were harmful or were not medically indicated (perhaps those who do not own such facilities don't order enough), but this finding raised the suspicions of congressmen and other regulators, and legislation is being developed that may prevent such arrangements in the future.[34] Even the American Medical Association (AMA) has changed its recommendations, now stating that physicians should not refer patients to testing facilities in which they have an ownership interest unless other arrangements would be impractical or detrimental to patients' health.[35]

"Unnecessary surgery" is often cited as an important factor in increased heath care costs. Rand Corporation studies in the early 1980s (based on retrospective chart reviews by panels of experts) are often cited as showing that one third of carotid endarterectomies performed were "unnecessary," based on criteria established by review of the peer literature. This statistic is then generalized to all surgical procedures, and the implication is made that medical costs would be easy to control if only all those doctors weren't merely trying to get rich. However, more recent studies of cardiac-related procedures indicate appropriate use of advanced techniques, with significant benefit for patients.[36–38] These studies demonstrate that less than 10% of the patients studied underwent inappropriate coronary bypass procedures. In addition, only 4% of the percutaneous coronary angioplasty procedures and coronary angiograms reviewed were felt to have been performed for improper indications. The authors further suggest that the percentage of unnecessary and uncertain procedures can be reduced even further as better data on outcomes are developed.

Out-of-pocket expenses for "unconventional medical services" are also an important source of health care spending.[39] These modalities, defined as

**THE CAUSES
OF INCREASED
HEALTH CARE COSTS**

OVERUTILIZATION BY
PROVIDERS
AND CONSUMERS

therapies not generally taught at medical schools in the United States, are used by patients with many chronic and common diseases such as cancer, arthritis, back pain, AIDS, and eating disorders. The treatments studied included acupuncture, chiropractic, and massage therapy. It is estimated that, in 1990, 425 million visits were made to providers of unconventional therapies at a cost of $13.7 billion, almost $10 billion of which was paid out of pocket. This amount was almost as much as the total out-of-pocket cost for all hospitalizations in the United States that same year.

Cataract surgery is also one of the areas mentioned most prominently by Congress and in the lay press when the issue of unnecessary services is discussed. Unsubstantiated figures of 20% to 30% are bandied about as estimates of the severity of the problem. However, objective data from the Office of the Inspector General reported to Congress in June of 1990 indicated that the figure is much lower. On the basis of information obtained from a study of the Peer Review Organization process in 10 states, the figure was placed at only 1.7%.[40]

Preliminary results of a study by the Johns Hopkins University School of Public Health also indicated low numbers of unnecessary procedures. Significant improvements in both vision and quality of life were found for most cataract surgery patients. When physical, visual, and psychological functions, as well as social participation, were considered, 95% of patients interviewed showed overall improvement. This figure is even higher than the 89% improvement rate published by the U.S. Department of Health and Human Services (HHS).[41]

OVERSUPPLY OF PHYSICIANS

It has been well documented that increasing the numbers of physicians increases health care costs, even when the actual income for each physician is lower.[42] This is true because the usual relationship between supply, demand, and determination of the cost of services generally applicable in the marketplace does not hold true for the delivery of medical care. Thus, an increase in the number of physicians actually results in an increase in the number of services rendered without lowering the cost per service. The reason is that physicians usually still control the choice of the type and number of services rendered, and patients at present have little incentive to quarrel because they are largely insulated from the cost of their treatment by third-party payors. It therefore follows that new physicians (ophthalmologists) will contribute to a significant increase in health care costs over the duration of their clinical careers.[43]

At present there are approximately 15,000 practicing ophthalmologists, an increase of one third compared with 10 years ago. It is projected that this number will rise to almost 20,000 in 2010.[44] There are presently approximately 1,461 residency positions available, including 457 first-year resident slots.[45] More than one half of these residents are below the age of 45, and many are women and minorities. Reducing the number of residents in training will be necessary if health care costs are to be controlled. This can be accomplished only by a concerted effort by those responsible for administering training programs, despite the antitrust risk that this course of action may entail.

IMPROVED TECHNOLOGY

Advances in medical technology have significantly increased the safety and effectiveness of many therapeutic and diagnostic procedures, but these advances have often been accompanied by significant cost increases. Many economists, health care theorists, and other gurus bemoan this development and long for a return to the old family physician and general practitioner, who is remembered as delivering kindly, hands-on, personal medical care.

However, it is clear that although this may be what Americans actually *need*, it is not really what many of them *desire*. These patients enjoy being scoped, scanned, CTed, and MRIed, and they come to the office familiar with and demanding these procedures. Woe be to the physician who does not comply! It's not that they don't want the other things; they simply want both.

As pointed out by Eli Ginsberg, the noted health economist,[46] Americans simply want continued access to more care and better care. At this point, at least, that means high-tech care, since often there are no viable alternatives. We lament the apparent increase in the use of life-prolonging medical technology on those with little chance of meaningful survival, and then pass laws such as the Americans with Disabilities Act that sometimes make it more difficult to discontinue that care. We marvel as tiny premature babies are kept alive and search the country to find donors for those who need life-saving transplants. We demand that those who are seriously ill with fatal diseases get experimental treatments (such as bone marrow transplants) even when the efficacy of the treatment is unknown. We spend billions on medical research and want to experience the fruits of those efforts as soon as they are available. We want the best, we want it now, and unfortunately we also want it to be inexpensive. Well, two out of three ain't bad; three out of three we just can't do!

Modern ophthalmology is a perfect example of the influence of high tech on a specialty and the increasing demand for the services it produces. Formerly the cryoprobe was all that was needed to remove a cataract (even I did not tumble lenses!); now we have available ingenious (and expensive) devices developed by talented ophthalmologists and engineers that can chop the cataract into tiny pieces to enable its removal through a much smaller incision. This advance, coupled with the transition to outpatient surgery, and other refinements in operative methods and lens implant technology have made rapid visual and functional recovery after cataract surgery the norm.

"Easy" cataract surgery, in turn, has made many older patients more willing to undergo the procedure. Patients who formerly "didn't want to go through it" are having second eyes done promptly and are also recruiting their friends and neighbors. Many of these patients benefit from the increased productivity and quality of life that follow, but the expense to society for this progress has been high, with over $3 billion being spent in the Medicare program alone. Too high? As someone who has witnessed first-hand the joy of patients who experience improved vision, I don't think so. However, those who make budget decisions for medical care in the future may not agree. We may have become too good for our own good.

Another example of the insatiable demand of Americans for high technology is the area of ophthalmic refractive surgery. Patients are willing to undergo radial keratotomy at a cost of thousands of dollars (mostly out of pocket) for the opportunity to see without glasses or contact lenses. There are long waiting lists for laser procedures designed to do the same thing, even though the efficacy, safety, and long-term consequences of the procedure are not yet completely understood.

The many tangible benefits of this improved technology have frequently been ignored, with only the cost being discussed. Patients now can return to work and most normal activities within a day or so after cataract surgery, instead of being forced to remain bedridden for weeks with sandbags surrounding their heads. Diabetics, formerly blind because of microvascular complications, remain productive employees, taxpayers, and parents because of spectacular advances in vitreous surgery. Lasers now allow treatment and prophylaxis of angle-closure glaucoma without the need for open eye surgery. Not many patients (or physicians, for that matter) really want to turn back the clock to the "good old days."

DEFENSIVE MEDICINE

Escalating professional liability expenses, added to the growing number and size of malpractice judgments, have led physicians to perform many tests and procedures of borderline value as a protection against subsequent litigation. A recent AMA study indicates that over 75% of physicians report that the threat of liability causes them to order studies they might otherwise consider unnecesssary.[47] This process, known commonly as "defensive medicine," adds significantly to the cost of medical care. Although accurate estimates of the cost are difficult to obtain, a recent study by the National Medical Liability Reform Coalition estimates the amount was at least $10 billion in 1991. This group, a coalition of physicians, hospitals, employers, and insurers, further estimates that $34 billion could be saved over 5 years if reform measures were instituted in 1994.[48] Other estimates[49] are even higher, with the expense for physician costs alone estimated at $15.1 billion in 1989.

STATE-MANDATED INSURANCE BENEFITS

The increase in state-mandated insurance benefits has driven up the cost for those companies willing to provide coverage for employees. This requirement for coverage of such services as chiropractic, acupuncture, homeopathic medicine, and other treatments of dubious value has added millions of dollars to the health care budget. It is reported that 16% of companies that provide no insurance do so because of the expense of mandates. Companies that use self-insurance for medical expenses are not subject to the mandates, and therefore more and more have chosen this method, which pays costs as incurred out of company revenue and does not depend on more traditional insurance protection. Since 1970, for example, 70% of companies with 1,000 or more employees and 30% of smaller companies chose self-insurance.[50]

DEMOGRAPHICS

Demographic considerations are also significant in the acceleration of health care expenditures, particularly at the federal level. The Census Bureau projects that, although the overall population growth rate of the United States is decreasing, the number of individuals aged 65 years and older will increase 26% between 1990 and the year 2010, reaching more than 39 million.[51] Because health care services are used more frequently as individuals age, this trend will dramatically affect expenditures. Older people spend more on health care than younger people, both in absolute terms and as a percentage of their total expenditures. Average Medicare expenses per person increase substantially as the age of the beneficiary increases. In 1987, $2,017 was expended for the group aged 65 to 74 years. In contrast, $3,215 was expended for those aged 85 years and older. Because these figures do not include the costs of long-term nursing home and custodial care, the actual bill for all health care in this age group is significantly higher.[52]

THE ADMINISTRATIVE BURDEN

To oversee the complex variety of health care plans available to the United States population, a large health care bureaucracy has evolved in both the federal government and the private health care industry (Fig. 2.8). An estimated 19% to 20% of the health care budget is spent on administrative expenses. The growth of costs in this area is at an even higher rate than that for medical expenses as a whole.

Although hard data are difficult to come by, HCFA estimated that the total price of administering health care in the United States, including overhead, profits, reserves, and insurance marketing, was $80 billion in 1991 (12% of all personal health expenses). The General Accounting Office (GAO) estimates that the cost was even higher, approaching 19% of total health care spending. On the basis of the data from HCFA, approximately half was spent on the costs associated with administration of private health insurance, government programs, and various health-related philanthropic organizations. The rest was spent on expenses associated with billing, half by hospitals and the remainder by physician and nonphysician providers.

Although it is often emphasized (especially by those who favor a single-payor form of universal health insurance coverage for the United States) that the overhead cost to *government* of administration and claims processing is much lower than that in the private sector, it is important to realize that this is so because many of the costs of complying with the regulations are shifted to the private sector, where they are assumed by hospitals and physicians.[53] These expenditures amount to almost $500 per capita—more than twice that paid in Canada, where administrative costs are only slightly over 10%. Even more revealing is the fact that administrative expenses in the United States increased by 37% in real dollars between 1983 and 1987. The reason for this is quite apparent when we consider the example of Blue Cross–Blue Shield of Massachusetts, which employs more workers to take care of 2.7 million subscribers than Canada's provincial health plans require to process more than 25 million individuals.[54]

Even more striking is the percentage of premium revenue that goes towards administrative expenses when small numbers of individuals (such as a typical small business) are insured. Recent studies estimate that *40% of premiums collected are used to cover nonmedical costs* such as commissions, marketing, billing and accounting, and general underwriting expenses. This is far in excess of the rate for companies with large numbers of employees (5.5%). Since the majority of companies in the United States fall into the small-firm category, this helps to explain the high costs incurred when these businesses attempt to purchase health care coverage for their employees.[55]

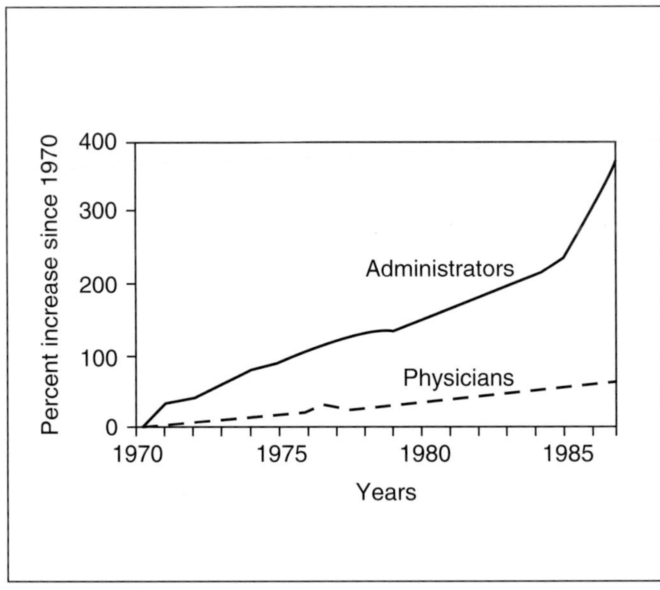

2.8 | Growth in administrators vs. physicians. (Adapted by permission from *N Engl J Med 1991; 324: 1255.*)

The expense and delays incurred in claim processing, reviews, and audits involving multiple vendors with dissimilar systems and standards have become a nightmare for patients and physicians alike. Private and public sector cost-containment procedures that involve multiple layers of review of medical decision-making by nonmedical personnel are cumbersome and are labor- and paperwork-intensive, with no clear evidence that they are effective in either containing costs or improving quality of care. They may, however, be detrimental to the ability of physicians to deliver appropriate, efficient medical care, and they have certainly altered the patient–physician relationship.

PATIENT ISOLATION FROM HEALTH CARE EXPENSES

One of the major difficulties with the present system of health insurance coverage is the isolation of patients from the true cost of their care. Most of the more than 130 million employees covered by employer-based plans have little incentive to minimize their medical expenses, since they are responsible for only a tiny fraction of the cost. Most patients are actually responsible for fewer out-of-pocket expenses than they were in the past (Fig. 2.9).

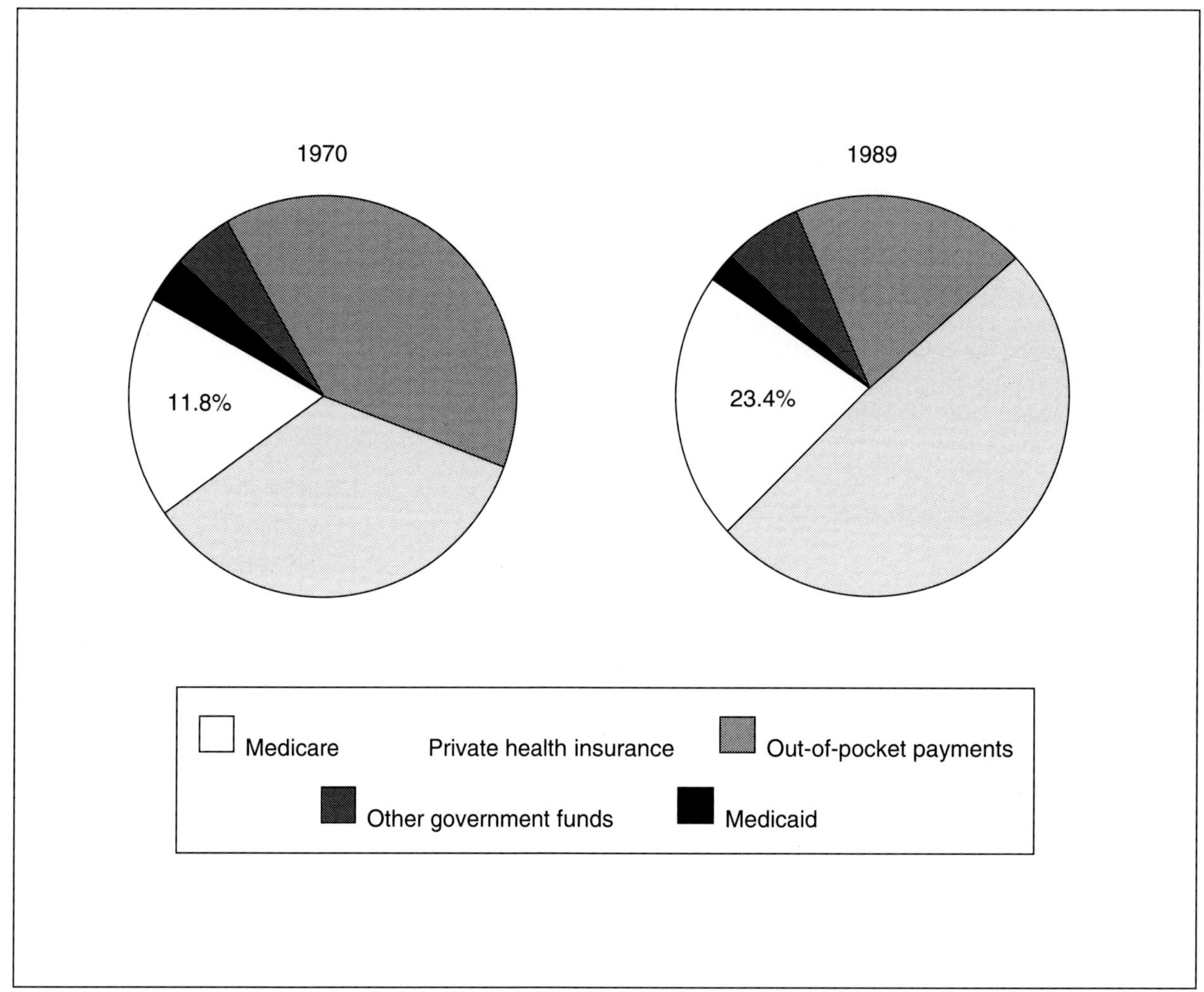

2.9 | Expenditures for physician services, by source of funds. (*Source:* Health Care Financing Administration, Office of National Cost Estimates. From PPRC, Report to Congress, 1993.)

Deductibles remain quite low (averaging only several hundred dollars in 1991), and after that most patients pay only a tiny percentage of the remaining charges. Office charges are also usually covered, except for a small co-payment. Therefore, patients have been insulated from the annual 12% to 15% cost increases that companies have had to face over the last decade.

Because they are so isolated from true costs, most patients do not discuss fees with physicians before obtaining treatment. Many (Fig. 2.10) also have no clue to what the cost might actually be. To increase employee interest in restraining health care expenses, many companies are significantly increasing the out-of-pocket contribution required before 100% coverage begins. They are also limiting the amount they will pay for certain tests and procedures (the patient pays the excess), and are giving the employee detailed fee and quality profiles for hospitals, physicians, and prescription drugs. Patients are encouraged to review fees with physicians and tell them that if they don't match the schedule they may go elsewhere. As one employee benefit manager put it, "We couldn't get their (employee) attention unless they had some substantial, personal financial involvement."[56]

FIGURE 2.10. Medical Mysteries: Consumer Estimates of Physician Fees

TYPE OF CARE	LOW ESTIMATE	HIGH ESTIMATE	AVERAGE ESTIMATE	ACTUAL COST*
Routine gynecological care and Pap smear	$ 8	$ 2,000	$ 320	$ 105
Complete physical	8	2,500	270	111
Adult office visit	3	200	151	47
Mammogram	10	4,000	315	88
Broken arm	10	3,800	583	418
Normal delivery of baby	45	80,000	2,595	1,999
Caesarean section delivery	200	70,000	3,661	2,636
Hysterectomy	100	45,000	3,048	2,493
Open-heart surgery	10	99,000	12,000	7,280

*National average fee.
Source: Wall Street Journal, February 8, 1993.

HEALTH CARE REFORM

BACKGROUND

As mentioned earlier, health care reform has become a primary concern of government, industry, and the citizenry in general. One of the reasons for this concerns the cost of health services. It is important, however, to keep cost figures in perspective. Although the United States spends more on health care, in both absolute and relative terms, than any other country (14% of GDP), the rate of increase in health care costs is actually not much higher than in many other countries (Fig. 2.11).[57] Since there is no "right" percentage of the GDP to spend on health care, it is also not surprising that the United States, with the world's largest per capita GDP, spends a significant proportion of that excess on health care. Americans consistently value quality of life as a major consideration, and (expensive) high-technology medicine has added significantly to that quality for many people. Lens implants, artificial joints, and coronary angioplasty have enabled many older citizens to remain active and productive far longer than in years past. In addition, if the GDP begins to grow and productivity increases as predicted, health care costs will shrink as a percentage of real income even if increases continue at the current rate.[58]

Another problem area derives from the lack of access to the system because of health insurance deficiencies (Fig. 2.12). In 1991 it was estimated that between 31 and 37 million individuals were uninsured, having no access to Medicare, Medicaid, or any other form of private health insurance. Of these, approximately 7 million were children under the age of 15 years, and just under 8 million were part-time workers employed for less than 18 hours per week. Most of the uninsured were not "poor"; the largest group had family incomes exceeding 185% of the poverty level. Almost one third of the uninsured were dependent children under the age of 24.

Sixteen million individuals were full-time employees (more than 18 hours per week) but had no insurance coverage. Of this group, 10% were self employed and just under 50% worked for small companies with less than 25 employees. If all employers were required to provide insurance for both employees and dependents, almost 80% of the uninsured would then be covered.

Many of those who have insurance are actually "underinsured" for possible catastrophic health care expenses, and few have coverage for long-term nursing home or custodial care.[59] Although patients worry greatly about

---

FIGURE 2.11. Per Capita Spending and Annual Average Change, 1980–1989

| | PER CAPITA SPENDING | | ANNUAL |
	1980	1989	AVERAGE CHANGE
United States	$1,059	$2,354	10.3%
Canada	806	1,683	10.6
Germany	749	1,232	4.3
Japan	515	1,035	5.7
France	656	1,274	10.8
United Kingdom	454	836	9.4

Source: AMA Advocacy Briefs, October 1991.

their ability to provide for themselves in their old age, recent attempts by Congress to provide catastrophic health care coverage for Medicare recipients were resoundingly defeated when the beneficiaries were asked to pay most of the cost. This supports the contention that although people in the United States are increasingly demanding greater and greater health care benefits, they are simply unwilling to pay for them.

Further evidence supporting this feeling is contained in the paradoxical responses to polls regarding health care in the United States. Most people state that they like their own physician but are dissatisfied with the health care system in general. They want to have the latest technology and facilities available even if they must pay higher taxes to do so. Those polled also believe that medical care should be available to all without regard to ability to pay, and almost two thirds feel that the United States spends too little on health care for those who cannot afford it themselves. However, only 22% are willing to pay an additional $200 in taxes to make this happen, a sum far below the actual amount needed to fund such programs.[60]

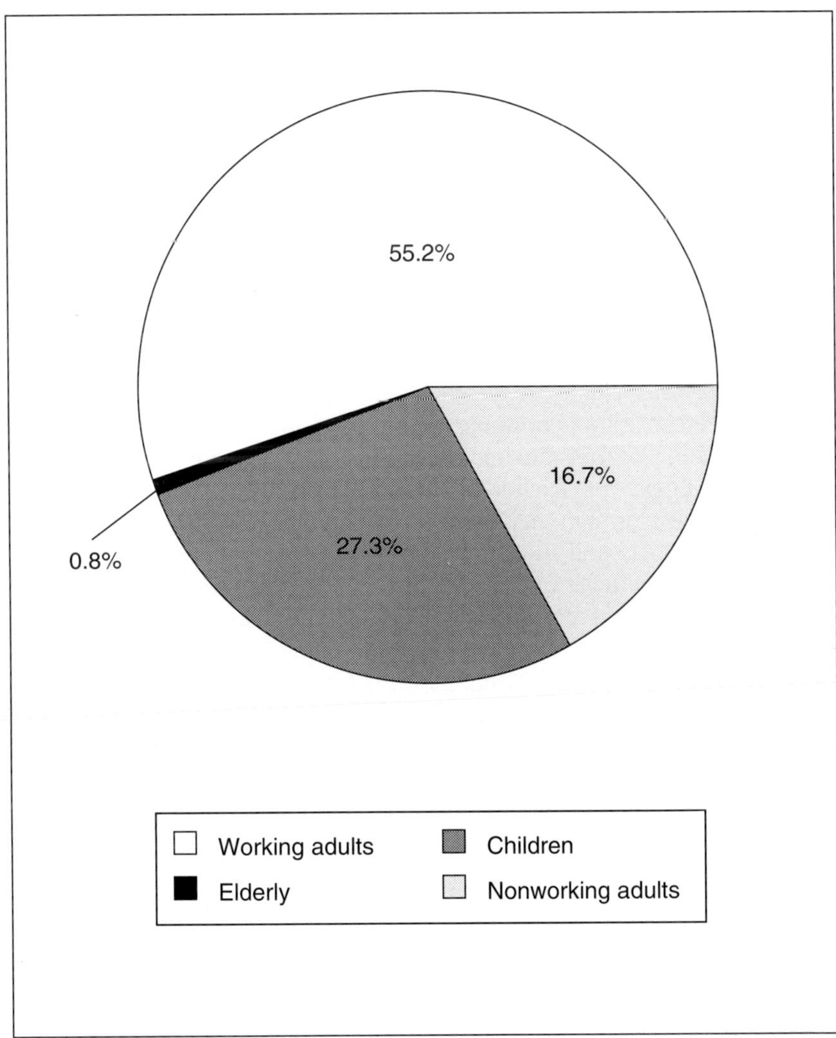

2.12 | Percentage of uninsured population in 1990. (*Source:* Employee Benefits Research Institute, Washington, D.C. From *Business and Health,* Mar 1992.)

There is also the question of whether we are really getting our money's worth from the system. Although we spend more than any other country in the world on health care, both in absolute terms and as a percentage of GNP, we still have high infant mortality and other indicators of less than optimal performance. However, in this context it is important to remember that we also have a host of social problems that increase health care costs but are not the fault of the health care system.

Violence in America is endemic. Children, women, minorities, and young people are most vulnerable. Firearms cause almost 900,000 nonfatal injuries yearly, and 500,000 emergency room visits each year are due to injury by violence. The homicide rate here is four times higher than that of Canada (the country with which we are most frequently compared), and violent assaults add $5.3 *billion* to direct health costs in the United States compared with $7.4 *million* in Canada.[61]

The infant mortality rate is steadily decreasing, although in the United States it is still higher than that of most of the other highly developed countries. However, these statistics are influenced by many factors not directly controlled by the health care system. The United States, for example, has many more low birth weight infants born to impoverished teenaged mothers who receive little prenatal care. Low birth weight is the primary cause of infant mortality within the first month of life. A high infant death rate is also linked to substance abuse, smoking, sexually transmitted infections, AIDS, and poor nutrition, all conditions prominent in many urban communities. These ills go beyond the power of medicine alone to correct.[62]

PERCEPTIONS OF THE CAUSES OF PROBLEMS

It is interesting and informative to consider the causes of and cures for the health care crisis in the United States as viewed by three distinct groups: patients, businessmen, and physicians. A review of recent polling data for the three groups is provided below.

PATIENTS

Almost three out of four consumers polled feel that overall health care costs are much too high. They cite high health insurance premiums, high costs of prescription drugs, inefficiency of the health care system, and physicians' desires to make a lot of money as the four main reasons for the high cost.[63] A recent Louis Harris poll indicated that one out of eight respondents had either been unable to get care or were refused care because they did not have insurance or could not afford it, and 30% postponed care because they could not afford it. This group believed overwhelmingly that the federal government should take the lead in seeing that all Americans have access to affordable health care. Furthermore, they felt that the government should achieve this end by controlling health insurance premium rates, prices of prescription drugs, and setting the rates that hospitals and physicians can charge for services.[64] Yet a third survey revealed that most prefer some sort of market reform over a national health insurance system.[65]

BUSINESS AND INDUSTRY

Because increasing health care costs continue to drag down earnings for both large and small corporations, business executives also have intense interest in health care reform. A recent survey of Fortune 500 CEOs[66] indicated that over 80% felt that "fundamental changes are needed in the system to make it work better." Almost 60% cited health care costs as a "major concern" for the company, and over half felt that government intervention was necessary. Many who were previously opposed to a system of national health insurance are now beginning to consider it as their only hope for reining in expenses. When a group of human resources executives (the new name for employment officers) was recently polled, they favored a federal policy to encourage managed care, along with government intervention to control costs, as the best mechanism for reform of the system.[67] Another group of business leaders also thought that instituting preventive health care programs, requiring second opinions and preadmission certification, and caps on medical malpractice awards would help to lower health costs.[68]

As one might expect, physicians also have views on the direction that health care reform should take. A national survey taken by *Medical Economics*[69] found that 80% of almost 5,000 physicians who responded believed that the health care system in the United States was in crisis. About half thought that it should be completely overhauled and that the job should be completed within 5 years. Most favored a mix of private and public payors. When asked their views regarding the cause of the health care problems, most believed that malpractice suits and insurance company administrative problems were the primary culprits (Fig. 2.13). They suggested that modifying the tort system and adopting standard insurance forms would go a long way towards solving the problem. They also favored capping drug costs, regionalization of hospital-based high-tech equipment, reducing patient demand for services, and restricting expensive care in terminal cases. Alterations of the fee structure for physicians, including paying for more preventative services, increasing financial incentives for primary care physicians, and decreasing payments for procedures by specialists were proposed by those (47%) who felt that physician fees were a major source of the problem.

PHYSICIANS

When rationing of resources was considered, most believed that priority should be given to infants and children. Almost two thirds felt that national health insurance was inevitable (down from 80% in 1971) but that all patients,

---

FIGURE 2.13. Major Contributors to Health Care Crises

FACTOR	PHYSICIAN RESPONSES PERCENT CITING
Malpractice suits	93%
Administrative costs	88%
Drug costs	86%
Hospital charges	85%
Patient demand	84%
Aging population	80%
"Unnecessary" care	75%
Too many specialists	51%

From *Medical Economics*, September 21, 1992, p. 64.

regardless of age, should contribute something unless they were unable to afford to do so. The majority favored contributions by both employers and employees, with a voucher system for those who were unemployed.

SOLUTIONS

It is likely that health care reform will occur in the next several years. The system that will emerge is not defined at this point, but it is expected that the large federal task force assembled in early 1993 will propose a plan that includes all Americans, regardless of income or employment status, and that makes some attempt to reduce costs. The proposed system will probably draw on elements from various systems that are presently in use, with the hope of combining the best components of the various plans into a hybrid that will satisfy most Americans. However, it is likely that no matter what system is chosen, costs will increase significantly and additional tax revenues will be required,[70] since elimination of unnecessary services and other sources of waste in the current system will not save enough money to finance care for those presently uninsured.

The stakes in the outcome of this process are enormous for health care providers. Therefore, it is not surprising that the health care industry makes sizable contributions to campaign funds for influential members of Congress and presidential candidates. In the 1990 election, the political action committee (PAC) sponsored by the American Academy of Ophthalmology was the second highest contributor in national elections, surpassed only by the AMA. Almost $1 million was spent, almost equally divided between Democrats and Republicans. This amount was almost three times the spending of the American Optometric Association and was also higher than the spending of the American Dental Association. The Academy PAC was also very active in 1992, ranking third in contributions as tabulated through midyear.[71]

There have been a multitude of proposals concerning the form of the new program. It is important that the final plan have certain characteristics. The features proposed by the executive editor of the *New England Journal of Medicine* include the requirement that it be *coherent*, in the sense that it can be easily understood by both patients and physicians. It should be *universal*, with no impediment to access for financial reasons, preexisting illness, or employment status. It should be structured in such a way that *costs* are *restrained* without the need for an unnecessarily burdensome surveillance system. The payment plan should also be *fair*, without excessive burdens on any single sector of the population, including business.[72] The key provisions described by the editor of *JAMA* are summarized in Fig. 2.14. Since the final product will draw from aspects of many systems presently in place, highlights of some of these are discussed below.

GOVERNMENT SPONSORED HEALTH INSURANCE
CANADA

The Canadian health care system is often touted as the ideal solution to our problems. It has provided health care at a lower cost than in the United States. The system, initiated in 1957, covers all residents in all provinces regardless of income, current health, or employment status. Each of the 10 provinces is charged with providing care that is comprehensive, accessible, and available from location to location within the country. Private insurance is forbidden to cover any benefits included in the basic package and is offered only for additional services such as dental care, nonprescription drugs, eyeglasses, and extended care. Initially, the system was funded with the promise that the federal government would pay half of all the costs for patient care during hospitalization. A similar stipulation was agreed to for physician services in 1968. Escalating costs, coupled with the recessionary economic climate in the 1970s, forced the government to abandon the open-ended 50–50 cost-sharing arrangement in 1977. The provinces since that time have found themselves saddled with the majority of health care costs, provoking a fiscal crisis in the system.[73]

At present the provinces pay almost 70% of the cost of health care, an amount that translates to almost one third of their total budgets. Because of the great antipathy of the majority of Canadians towards user fees for health care, the province of Ontario has tried to limit costs by reducing covered benefits for the 10 million people in its health care system. It has also capped spending on health care at $16.9 billion, an increase of only 2% over last year compared with the average annual increases of 11.2% that occurred during the 1980s. The fee schedule for physicians was increasd by only 1.75%, and hospitals had an increase of only 1%. As the number of covered services is reduced, it is anticipated that private insurance will be used by many individuals to cover these costs, reducing the overall drain on the public sector.[74]

Physicians are paid on a "fee for service" basis (they are not government employees) based on a negotiated fee schedule. No balance billing is allowed. Since there is only one payor, the process of reimbursement is relatively streamlined and administrative costs are low. Although Canada has more active physicians and uses more services per capita than the United States, overall payments to physicians are less because of strict fee controls. This enables Canada to keep costs down without the strict utilization review programs that are prevalent in the United States.[75]

Hospitals operate under an entirely different system. They have separate operating and capital budgets controlled by each province. For day-to-day operations, each hospital receives a fixed sum on a yearly basis. This plan is designed to encourage them to cut costs and use funds efficiently. Sometimes, however, the push to cut expenses produces undesirable consequences, such as attempting to fill beds with low-cost long-term care patients to prevent the admission of more expensive acutely ill ones. Hospitals also

---

FIGURE 2.14. The Grid Upon Which to Test Health Care Reform Proposals

Does the proposal achieve the following:
Provide access to basic medical care for all of our people?
Produce real cost control?
Promote continuing quality?
Limit professional liability?
Reduce administrative hassle?
Retain necessary patient and physician autonomy?
Consider long-term care?
Encourage primary care?
Enhance disease prevention?
Possess staying power after 5, 10, or 20 years?

From *JAMA*, October 21, 1992, p. 2.82.

decrease costs by delivering services of lower intensity due to budgetary limitations on equipment, supplies, and available labor.[75]

Capital expenses are also strictly controlled. The Ministries of Health control spread of new technologies and equipment through tight restrictions on the availability of funds for these purposes. This results in the availability of fewer specialized and high-technology services per person than in the United States (Fig. 2.15), and has led to the development of long waiting periods for some high-technology specialty care services (Fig. 2.16). Aside from the anxiety that such a situation produces, the patient's health may deteriorate during the waiting period or other more risky procedures may be substituted. The situation became so desperate at one point during 1990 that the Ministry of Health of British Columbia was forced to negotiate contracts with hospitals in the state of Washington to provide cardiac surgical services for over 700 patients.[76]

How does this all balance out? It is apparent that Canada continues to spend a lower percentage of its GDP on medical services than the United States. However, the rate of increase in spending on health-related services in

2.15 | Availability of selected medical technologies. (From GAO Report, HRD-91-90, p. 50.)

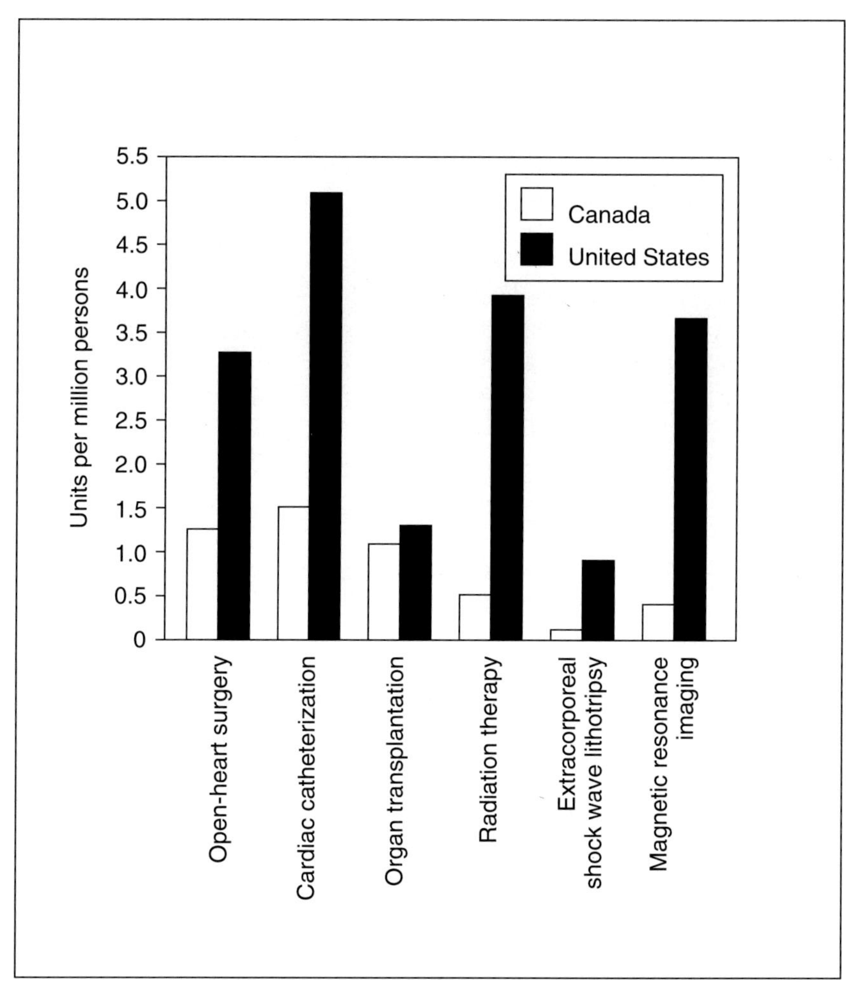

recent years has approached that of the United States, and the provincial budgets are being increasingly burdened by rising health care costs. The system provides excellent primary care and has no financial barriers to access. Administrative costs are lower, but this is due in part to primitive utilization review and budgetary processes that do not provide sufficient data to allow improved eficiency in the future. Development of new high technology is virtually nonexistent, and the system depends on the United States as a backup in some situations.

Would it work in the United States? Obviously, no one knows for certain, but there are significant barriers to implementation. The first is related to demographic considerations. The United States is 10 times more populous and geographically much less compact. Our population is older, and we have significantly more poverty, AIDS, violence, teenaged pregnancy, and urban slums, all of which increase health costs significantly. Our tolerance for longer waiting periods for tests such as MRIs, CT scans, and mammograms has not yet been assessed. The adequacy of the bureaucratic systems in place to handle the administrative load of being single-source payors for all citi-

---

FIGURE 2.16. Queuing for Specialty Care Services in Ontario (October 1990)

	NUMBER OF PROGRAMS REPORTING QUEUES	NUMBER OF PATIENTS WAITING		NUMBER OF DAYS WAITING	
		MINIMUM	MAXIMUM	MINIMUM	MAXIMUM
CT SCAN					
Emergent	0 of 13	0	0	0	0
Urgent	4 of 13	6	15	1	21
Elective	13 of 13	40	1,200	2	180
MRI					
Emergent	1 of 7	1	1	2	2
Urgent	2 of 7	75	75	3	30
Elective	7 of 7	100	893	1	480
Cardiovascular surgery					
Emergent	0 of 10	0	0	0	0
Urgent	7 of 10	4	87	1	30
Elective	9 of 10	11	263	7	180
Eye surgery					
Emergent	0 of 9	0	0	0	0
Urgent	3 of 9	1	1	1	14
Elective	9 of 9	10	400	30	360
Orthopedic surgery					
Emergent	0 of 8	0	0	0	0
Urgent	6 of 8	6	12	14	30
Elective	8 of 8	17	380	60	360

Source: GAO Report, HRD 91–90, p. 55.

zens has not been evaluated. Moreover, can these same bureaucrats, unsuccessful in the past in restraining the escalation of health care costs in the Medicare and Medicaid systems, suddenly develop the expertise to do so in a single-payor system?

GERMANY

The German system of health insurance was begun in 1883 by Otto von Bismarck as an attempt to quell social unrest among the working class and to decrease the power of the labor unions. It has evolved into a system that today insures almost 90% of all citizens through a system of "sickness funds." At present there are approximately 1,147 of these organizations, many of which are associated with private employers. All workers with an income of less than $36,580 must contribute to the sickness fund responsible for paying for their care. The contribution varies from 8% to 16% (average 13%) of salary with the employer and employee each paying an equal share, without reference to state of health or number of dependents. Retirees and the unemployed are also covered and receive identical benefits. The premiums collected by these funds are then distributed to physicians who are paid on a fee-for-service basis according to a negotiated payment schedule. Hospital-based physicians are compensated by salaries based on specialty and experience. Hospitals receive their operating expenses from the sickness funds and capital budgets are financed primarily by the state. Private insurance is purchased by about 10% of the population, with benefits that are essentially similar to those provided by the sickness funds.[77]

Germans pay about 9% of their GDP for health care while providing virtually universal coverage and avoiding many of the delays and limits on high-tech procedures that characterize the Canadian system. Cost control is a major issue and fees are tightly regulated by the funds, which have tied the rate of rise of health care costs to the overall rate of rise of workers' wages. If volume of services increases, the "conversion factor" used to determine fees is reduced, thus keeping fees within the global budget. Utilization review techniques are well developed, and profiles are available to compare individual physicians with their peers. Those who exceed the standards may find their reimbursement reduced and some are actually asked to return funds to the system.[78]

Despite the tight controls on the German system, costs continued to spiral upwards during 1991. In January of 1993 additional limits on drug charges were introduced and dentists' fees were reduced. Larger co-payments for some services were instituted, and hospitals were shifted from a per-diem reimbursement (which was widely abused) to a diagnosis-based system. Plans are also in the works to institute HMOs and other managed care systems later in this decade.[79]

BRITAIN

The British system is a true cradle-to-grave national health service system that provides universal coverage for all citizens. Outpatient and hospital care are included, along with prescription drugs (with a small co-payment). The system is financed through general taxation via the National Health Service and by employer and employee payments to a National Insurance Fund. Approximately 10% of patients have private insurance, which allows then to bypass the long NHS waiting lists that exist for many elective procedures. This option has in effect sanctioned the creation of a true two-tiered system.

Britain, too, has been faced with rising health care costs and the need to better utilize its resources. It has allowed certain hospitals to become self-governing trusts and has demanded that they compete for income by contracting with general physicians and other hospitals for the opportunity to provide patient services. In addition, practitioners who have more than 11,000 patients are given a fixed sum of money to purchase the hospital services used in the care of their patients.[80]

JAPAN

Japan is a country with a population of 122 million individuals in an area the size of Montana. Most of the people live in densely populated urban areas and are ethnically very homogeneous. The entire population is covered by universal insurance in a single-tier system, with 60% being enrolled in programs sponsored by employers and 30% in government-sponsored national health insurance. The remainder are covered by a geriatric plan for those over the age of 75. Co-payments are prominent in both systems, with contributions of up to 30% being required for some services. About 6.8% of the GDP is spent on the provision of health care.

Physicians are reimbursed on a uniform fee schedule regardless of the type of plan involved. Low fees encourage frequent brief visits, which are not always consistent with quality care. Capital expenses for hospitals and equipment are not heavily regulated, with the result that the country has the highest number per capita of CT scanners in the world. The government (as in Germany) heavily regulates the price of pharmaceuticals, and the charge for an MRI scan is only $177. Administrative costs are quite low because of the single-fee schedule, and malpractice suits are rare.[81]

The direct contribution of corporations to health care premiums for employees and dependents is quite small compared with that of the United States ($700 versus $3,452 in the same year). This represents about 2.7% of wages and is matched by the employee. This relatively low contribution is intentional, because there is strong belief in all quarters that the government should protect the economy by keeping employer contributions as low as possible. Unlike many American companies, Japanese corporations are also not responsible for health care costs for retirees, resulting in significant savings.[82]

Physicians derive a significant portion of their income from dispensing drugs. As a result, the Japanese spend more on drugs than any other nation. Almost 30% of the country's total health budget is spent on drugs (as opposed to 7% in the United States), and it is estimated that many hospital admissions are precipitated by drug reactions. Newer, more expensive drugs are prescribed frequently, even when there are no clear-cut theraputic advantages, because profit margins are higher. The government has tried to control the process by switching to a Diagnosis Related Group (DRG) payment system with a fixed monthly drug budget based on the medical diagnosis.[83]

OTHER HEALTH CARE REFORM SUGGESTIONS FOR THE UNITED STATES

MANAGED COMPETITION

This model of health care reform (the "Jackson Hole Plan") is based on a structure that integrates government regulation with free market competition (Fig. 2.17). It unites individuals, small employers, and other purchasers of health care benefits into large networks to bid for services from organized groups of health care providers (Fig. 2.18). These providers would be forced to offer a standard package of benefits (the mandates to be determined by a government panel), so that only price and quality would have to be considered by the buyer. Employers would purchase care for their employees and the unemployed would have the premium paid from general tax revenues. Individuals could not be excluded because of health status or preexisting medical conditions. It is hoped that limitations on the tax deductibility of employer contributions would encourage both employees and employers to pay close attention to price, since any excess would count either as taxable income to the employee, or as a non-tax-deductible expense to the employer.[84,85]

Market forces, rather than global budget limits, represent the principle

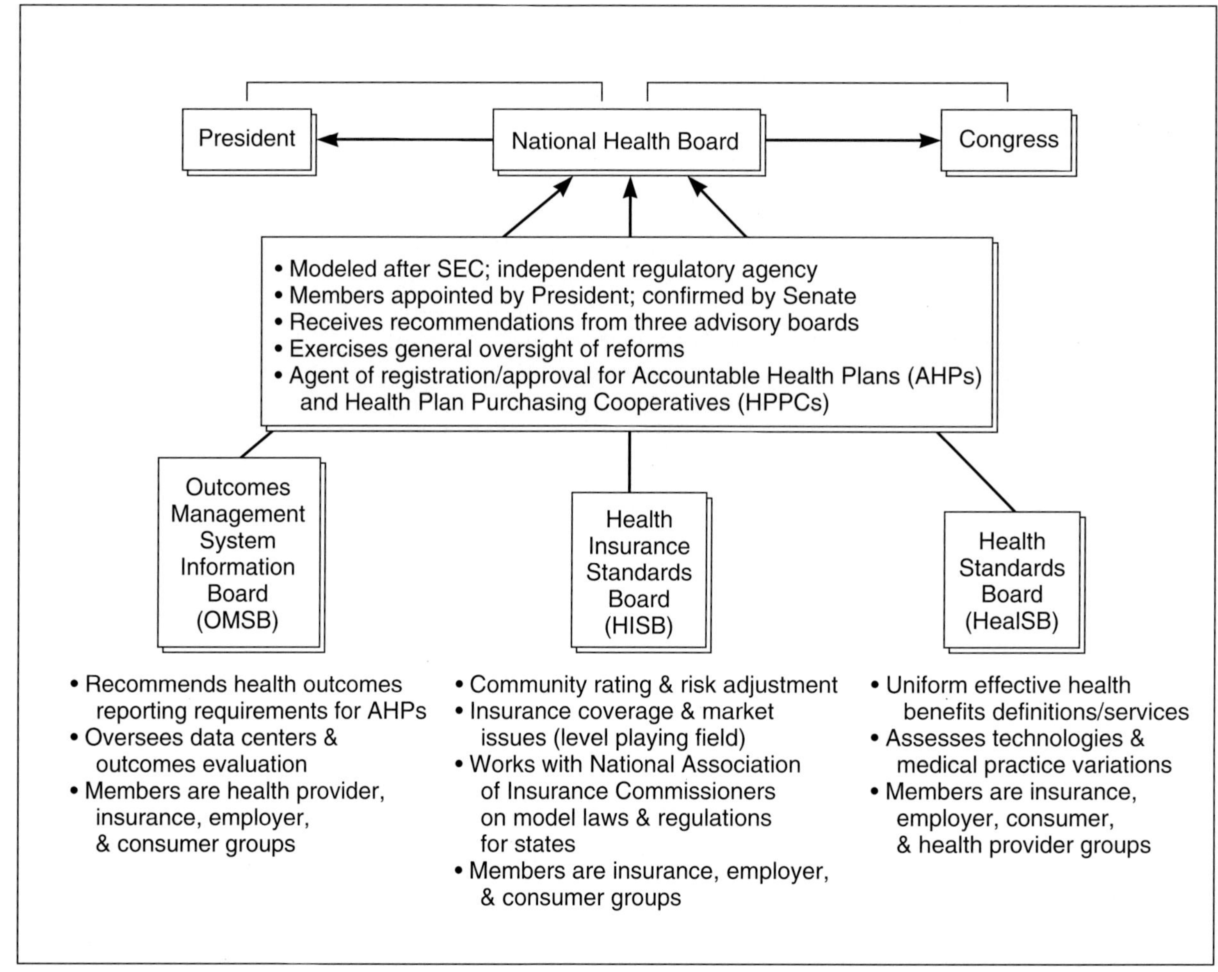

2.17 | Managed competition: National Health Board and private sector advisory boards. (*Source:* The Jackson Hole Group Proposals, Sept 1991.)

mechanisms for cost containment. The California Public Employees' Retirement System (CALPERS) represents the prototype of this system. Covering 887,000 individuals, it uses its buying clout to negotiate rates with various insurers throughout California, and has recently been successful in keeping its rate of premium growth below both previous increases and the national average. Unhappy with the cost of care purchased from its largest insurer (the Kaiser Permanente system) CALPERS responded by restricting new enrollment in the plan and eventually forced a rate reduction from the HMO for 1993. Co-payments for office visits and prescription drugs, which formerly were not employed extensively by Kaiser, became an important part of cost and utilization control for the plan, so that overall costs were not actually reduced very much.[86,87] The federal government, through the Federal Employee Health Benefit Program covering over 9 million individuals, also has a similar program.[88] Various states (for example, Florida), and other large employee groups are also developing similar systems.[89–91]

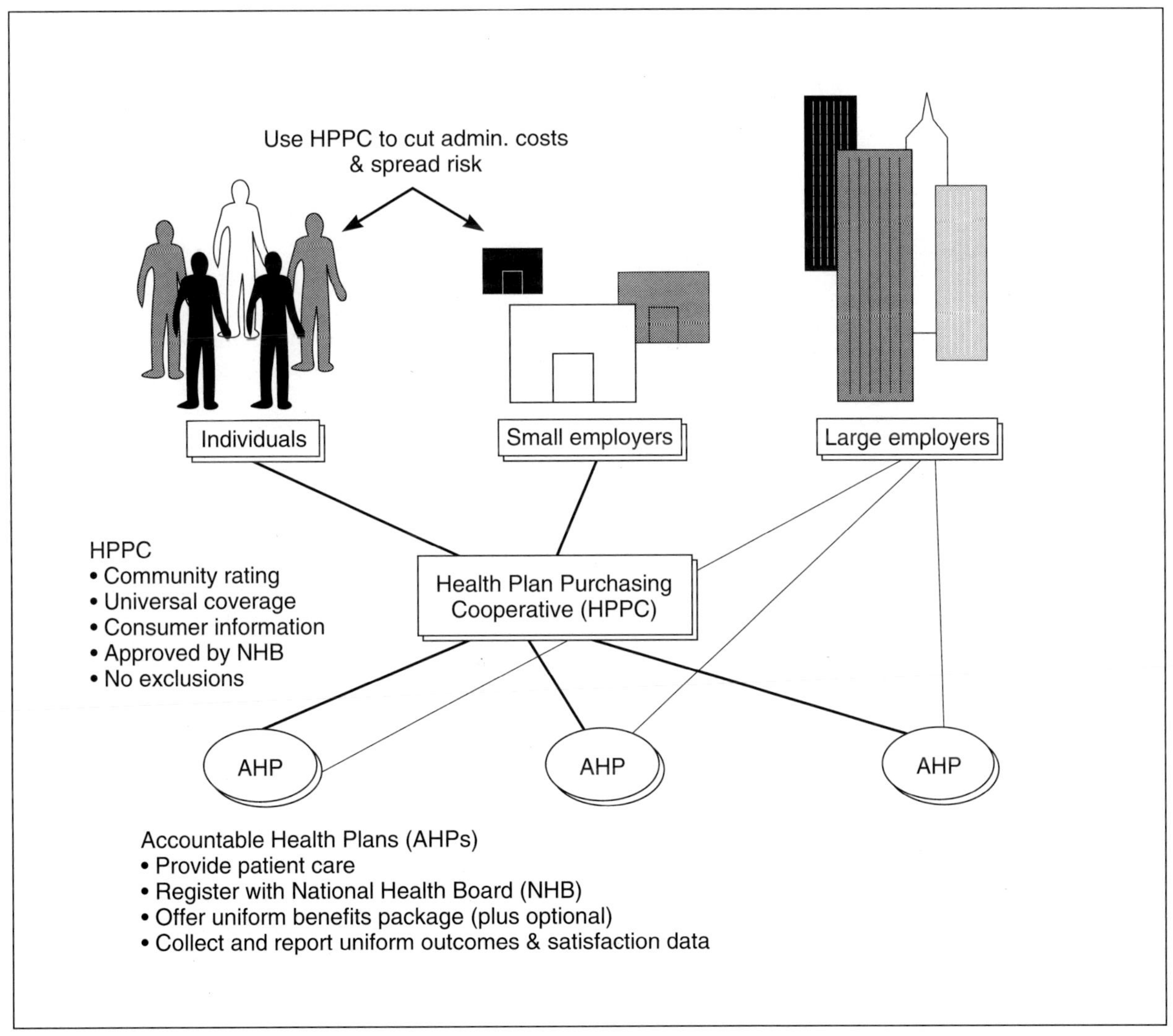

2.18 | Managed competition. (*Source:* The Jackson Hole Proposal, Sept 1991.)

Not everyone believes that managed competition represents the most viable option for health care reform. The National Leadership Coalition for Health Care Reform, a diverse organization that includes representatives from industry, unions, and consumer groups, feels that implementation will take too long and expenditures will continue to rise.[92] There are concerns that medical costs cannot be controlled in an open-ended price competitive market, and that quality may suffer if decisions are made primarily by third-party payors rather than physicians.[93] The program also may not work well in rural areas, where populations are too small to support true competition.[94] Some analysts feel that the success claimed by CALPERS was due in large part to budget caps imposed in California because of the fiscal crisis in the state.[95] Still, at the present time, managed competition, with the possible addition of global budget caps, remains the favorite program of the Clinton administration.[96]

AMERICAN MEDICAL ASSOCIATION: "HEALTH CARE AMERICA"

This program, sponsored by the AMA, has as its cornerstones universal coverage, cost containment, quality, and freedom of choice.[97] The proposal suggests that employers be required to provide health care coverage to employees and dependents, and expansion of the federal Medicaid program. It would foster competition by requiring providers to release price information, and insurers would be forced to reveal what they would pay for medical services. Cost containment would also be achieved by removing state-mandated health care benefits, reducing administrative expenses with standard claim forms and electronic billing systems, and implementing professional liability reforms. It would encourage the development of practice parameters to ensure that only appropriate services are provided, and would encourage emphasis on preventive services and healthy lifestyles. Most of all, it would preserve the freedom of individual consumers to obtain services from the physician, hospital, and health care plan that best meets their needs.

"PLAY OR PAY"

The "play or pay" option involves requiring employers either to pay for health insurance for employees or to contribute additional taxes into a fund (Americare) to provide insurance paid for by the federal government. Although the actual cost of the proposal is not known, it is likely that the initial tax increase for those businesses choosing to "pay" would be 7% to 9% of payroll. There is concern that this increase may force some small employers to lower wages, decrease hours (to make some employees part-timers), or even eliminate jobs altogether. The Employee Benefits Research Institute projects that a 9% payroll tax will cost 1 million jobs.[98] Another potential obstacle is that companies whose health care costs exceed the amount of the proposed tax would have no incentive to "play." They would simply "pay" to place their employees in the public system. According to Labor Department estimates, this would eventually lead to approximately half of the population being included in the public system, a prelude to a true single-payor national health insurance system. In addition to institutional opposition from the AMA,[99] others in industry also voice concerns (aside from the costs involved) that this central bureaucratic control will stifle innovation, research, and medical education.[100]

There are those who favor a single-payor national health insurance system for the United States. These plans would provide coverage for all Americans, sponsored through tax-funded federal- and state-directed programs. PNHP is essentially a transplant of the Canadian system.[101] Health USA would involve a single payor but would also incorporate many of the aspects of managed competition discussed earlier.[102]

HEALTH USA AND PHYSICIANS FOR A NATIONAL HEALTH PROGRAM (PNHP)

Traditionally, health care in the United States has been financed by "indemnity" type of health insurance. Under this system, patients choose a physician, obtain diagnostic services and treatment from the physician, and then are billed. The patient purchases insurance to pay all or part of the cost but is ultimately responsible for all charges. Fees are determined by the physicians and the other entities that provide the services, usually with few restrictions. Patients typically have free choice of physicians and physicians have access to all patients with insurance. Income is truly based on "fee for service," and there are few restraints on the number and type of services rendered. The greater the number and intensity of services, the more revenue generated.

MANAGED CARE

This method of payment of health care costs is regarded as inflationary and is also historically biased in favor of procedural rather than cognitive services. Because the benefits are essentially unlimited, the cost of providing indemnity insurance has skyrocketed and is now beyond the reach of most corporations and other entities that provide benefits for employees.[103] These institutions have therefore sought alternative forms of paying for health care services, and it is because of this stimulus that the various forms of managed care have developed.

The general term "managed care" encompasses a variety of programs that have as their common characteristic the integration of payment for and delivery of appropriate medical services in a carefully regulated system designed primarily to curtail costs. Features common to most of the programs include restriction of physician choice, discounted or capitated fee payments, financial risk sharing by physicians, and strict utilization and quality control provisions usually administered by nonphysicians.

A cogent analysis by the Jackson Hole Group[104] outlines some of the serious inherent deficiencies of many current managed care systems. The analysis points out that the present programs increase administrative complexity without necessarily increasing quality of care and that they encourage payors, physicians, and insurers to manipulate the system for their own benefit. Fragmentation of markets and exclusionary underwriting practices also limit the efficiency of many private programs and fail to protect many patients from financial disaster caused by extended illness. Most importantly, the present systems fail to encourage thoughtful, informed medical decision making based on outcomes analysis and other available scientific data. In addition, it is not even clear, in many instances, that the savings claimed by those who favor the present systems actually exist.[105]

The variety of managed care programs available seems almost endless, with new strategies and hybrids being introduced frequently. Some of the more commonly encountered types are defined in Figure 2.19. They fall into

---

FIGURE 2.19. Glossary of Terms

Exclusive provider organization (EPO): A smaller version of an HMO. Subscribers are eligible to receive services only from participating providers. There is no deductible; the patient must pay a predetermined copayment for each service. Patients who go outside the network might not be reimbursed for those health care costs.

Fee-for-service: An arrangement under which patients pay doctors, hospitals, or other health care providers for each service rendered. Most then seek reimbursement from a private insurer or the government.

Gatekeeper or primary care physician: The individual designated by the plan to control the member's access to the system's services and providers.

Health maintenance organization (HMO): A pre-paid health care plan under which people enroll by paying a set annual fee. They then receive all the medical services they need through a group of affiliated doctors and hospitals, often with no additional co-payments or fees.

Independent practice association: A type of HMO that contracts with individual physicians to provide services to the HMO's enrollees. Doctors maintain their own private practices and thus can contract with other HMOs or see regular fee-for-service patients as well.

Managed care: A general term for organizing networks of health care providers, such as doctors and hospitals, to enhance the cost effectiveness of their work. An HMO is a common form of managed care.

Medicare: The federal program providing health insurance for people aged 75 and older and for disabled people of all ages.

Open vs. closed panels: An open panel permits virtually all physicians to contract with the managed care plan to provide services. A closed panel does not permit all physicians to become part of the provider network.

Physician/hospital organizations (PHO): A joint venture between a hospital and private practices to offer managed care plans or to contract to provide services to independent subscribers.

Point of service (POS): A managed care plan combining an HMO's control of costs with a PPO's more liberal policy of allowing patients to select providers. If the patient stays within the network, the primary care physician manages all the care, and the patient incurs little or no out-of-pocket costs. Patients who obtain care outside the network pay a higher deductible and coinsurance; typically they are reimbursed for about 75% of non-network costs.

Preferred provider organization (PPO): An arrangement under which an insurance company or employer negotiates discounted fees with networks of health care providers in return for guaranteeing a certain volume of patients. Enrollees in a PPO can elect to receive treatment outside the network but have to pay higher copayments or deductibles for it.

Sources: Wall Street Journal, March 11, 1993, p. A12, and *Argus,* March 1993, p. 21.

two general types: capitated (HMO) and modified fee for service (PPO). Some health care analysts believe that these types of plans reduce health care expenditures, although the evidence available is not always convincing. In 1991, according to benefits company A. Foster Higgins, the cost to employers for HMO coverage was 14% less than that for indemnity coverage, with costs for PPOs about 6% less.[106] On the other hand, twice as many employers interviewed by the Health Insurance Association of America (HIAA) felt that HMOs were "not at all successful" in controlling rising health care costs as those that felt they were "very successful." Most felt that they were "somewhat successful."[107] Enrollment in 20 of the largest HMO organizations increased by 28% in 1992. Since the rate of increase in HMO premiums is continuing to moderate (Fig. 2.20), it is likely that enrollment will continue to climb.[108]

According to *Medical Economics*, the typical physician grossed 30% more from HMOs and PPOs in 1991 than in 1989. Plan participation has

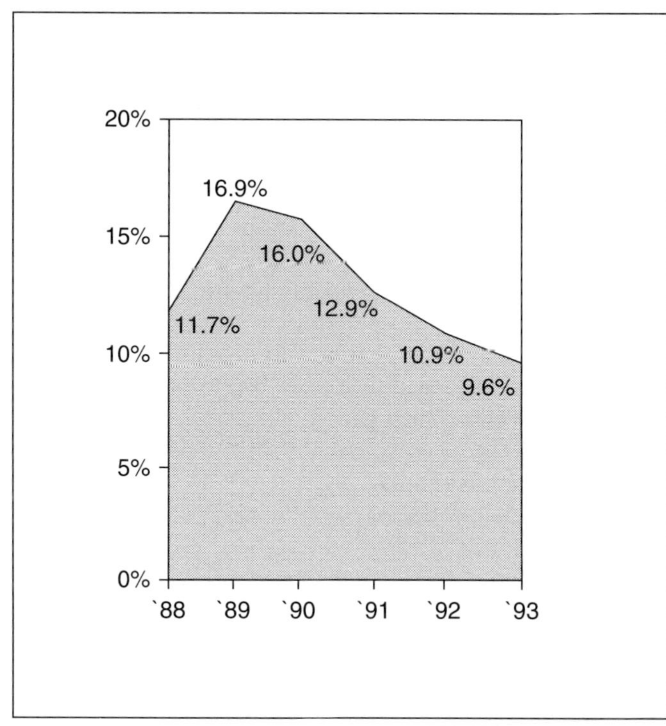

2.20 | Average HMO premium increases, 1988–1993. (*Source: American Medical News,* Dec 28, 1993, p. 14.)

increased, although half of those interviewed still belong to neither an HMO nor a PPO. Large groups are much more likely to participate than solo practitioners. Less than 10% of the ophthalmologists were members of more than five plans, but over 50% belonged to at least one. Most derived less than 10% of their income from the plans.[109]

It is likely that ophthalomologists will find an increasing need to participate in various types of managed care programs (including the provision of capitated care) to maintain adequate access to patients. Many patients will find themselves unable to continue care with their present ophthalmologist because the physician is not a member of the panel chosen by the carrier. In this situation, if patients wish to retain their present ophthalmologists, they will have to pay either the entire bill out of pocket or pay an increased co-payment and/or deductible as a penalty for using an out-of-plan physician. This form of economic blackmail forces patients to make difficult choices, because many are unable to afford the additional cost associated with the desire to choose their own physicians.

Even more alarming is the fact that some patients with eye pathology may be unable to see an ophthalmologist at all unless an optometrist decides that additional consultation is required. This system is based on the idea that optometry is less costly than ophthalmology for providing "routine" care and therefore is more cost effective over the long haul, a hypothesis that has certainly not been supported by reliable and reproducible data. Nevertheless, many plans still place the optometrist in the ophthalmologic "gatekeeper" role, with control over subsequent referrals to various medical specialties, including ophthalmology.

Primary care physicians, the "gatekeepers" for medical services in many managed care plans, are often under significant *economic* pressure not to refer "routine" patients directly to specialists, and in some cases may not even have that option available. This conflict arises because the cost for the patient evaluation by the specialist may be deducted from the pool from which the primary care physician is compensated, whereas the cost of seeing an optometrist may not. There is a temptation, therefore, to simply send the patient to the optometrist and allow the decision for additional referral to be made there.

With the trend towards groups of physicians organizing to bid on managed care contracts involving large numbers of patients, the solo practitioner must be flexible and must consider less conventional practice arrangements. Many will find it necessary to organize into larger groups to bid for patient care contracts. Capitated contracts, in particular, must be carefully evaluated to be certain that the amount of care to be delivered is adequately compensated for by the capitation rate.[110] Detailed suggestions on the evaluation of various types of managed care arrangements are discussed in Chapter 5.

VISION CARE PLANS

Designed primarily to provide routine refractive care, vision care plans often make it difficult for ophthalmologists to be part of their provider panels because many are sponsored by optometric organizations. In an attempt to maintain patient access, ophthalmologists in some parts of the country have formed networks that market vision care services directly to third-party payors and large companies. Although the reimbursement from vision care programs for refractive services is, in general, lower than normal office charges, many ophthalmologists accept this in return for maintaining access to the patient for medical services and also for products, such as contact lenses and glasses, that can serve as additional profit centers.

Formation of a Federal Cataract PPO for Medicare patients, modeled after that developed for coronary artery surgery, has been championed by HCFA as a cost-saving measure. The intent is to limit cost by including the preoperative tests, physician fee, facility fee, implant cost, and all followup care in a total package. Because of the potential danger that the program presents for Medicare patients, the American Academy of Ophthalmology filed a lawsuit to enjoin HCFA from pursuing the project.[111] This legal challenge has been unsuccessful so far (an initial loss in court is being appealed), and recently HCFA awarded contracts to groups in Cleveland, Dallas, and Phoenix as part of its pilot project. The bids ranged from $2,194 to $2,513. It is estimated that 15,000 patients will be treated during the 3-year pilot period.[112] It is ironic (but not entirely surprising) that the government is proposing a program based on lower charges per procedure, with income to be sustained by increased volume, at the same time that it accuses ophthalmologists of performing too many cataract extractions! It can be hoped that this project, which was favored by the Bush administration, will disappear under new leadership at HHS.

CATARACT PPO

A new program for Medicare beneficiaries, Medicare Select, has been developed in 10 states to reduce the cost of supplemental insurance. This plan is intended to decrease by up to 20% the premium paid by beneficiaries for their Medigap policies by placing them in an HMO. These policyholders will receive full benefits as long as they use providers who are in the network for routine medical care.[113] This joint effort of the insurance industry and the government could serve as a model for future cooperative efforts to make health care costs more affordable.

A similar program for Medicaid patients is also being tested. This approach is being used by states desperate to control the increasingly unpredictable escalation of costs for indigent health care. Participation rates range from 1% to 100% in states such as Arizona and Utah. Overall, about 3.6 million individuals, accounting for about 12% of the total Medicaid population, will be enrolled.

HHS endorses the process because it believes that savings will accrue from decreased use of hospital tests, x-rays, lab tests, and drugs. Problems with fraud and abuse that plagued similar programs in the past have presumably been corrected with better contract language and oversight capabilities. It is especially hoped that use of preventive services, such as prenatal visits and immunizations, will be increased.[114]

MEDICARE AND MEDICAID HMOS

The state of Orgeon, in an attempt to ensure universal access to health care for all of its residents, has established a plan that has as its major cost-containment provision a controversial proposal to ration health care by limiting benefits. Under the plan, fewer services would be offered to those on Medicaid but no one in Oregon would be without coverage for any of those services. The state essentially performed a cost–benefit analysis on 709 services previously reimbursed under the Medicaid system, ranking them by medical effectiveness and contribution to society. Initially the state decided that it could afford to cover approximately 587 of these services, but this number was modified after the conditions were regrouped to address concerns about violations of the Americans with Disabilities Act, and at present 568 services qualify for payment under the program. The procedure that ranked first overall was treatment of a severe head injury, with treatment of a sebaceous cyst bringing up the rear. Some controversial conditions, such as treatment

THE OREGON MEDICAID PLAN: HEALTH CARE RATIONING BY STATUTE

of anencephalic infants and liver transplantation for those with alcoholic cirrhosis, were included after being denied initially. Hospice and care for low birth weight infants were also late additions.[115] When objections were raised that the program amounted to rationing care, those in favor of this concept remarked that care is currently rationed (according to whether or not the patient has insurance), and that this system will be inherently more fair since all low-income individuals will derive at least some benefits.

The basic package of covered services includes preventive care and covers most major diseases that affect women and children. It also adds dental coverage, prescription drugs, routine physical examinations, and almost every type of transplant. The coverage package has been extended to include all residents who fall below the federal poverty level, as well as children and pregnant women with slightly higher incomes. The working uninsured will have to be covered by employers in 1995, using the program as a guide for minimal benefits that must be provided. High-risk pools and a small business insurance package are also being developed.

The initial attempts by Oregon to obtain a waiver of HHS regulations to implement the plan was blocked by the Bush administration, ostensibly because of concerns that the original rankings took into account the quality of life of the patient in violation of the Americans with Disabilities Act. The Clinton administration, in March of 1993, gave permission for implementation of the program as a 5-year pilot project after imposing additional safeguards. At present it is proposed that the additional cost of the plan, which is expected to exceed $100 million by the time the project is completed, be covered by a provider tax on hospitals, dentists, and physicians, since they will receive added income from reimbursements. Additional revenue would come from increased taxes on alcohol and cigarettes.[116]

PHYSICIAN PAYMENT REFORM

It is difficult to predict how all the aforementioned trends will affect the practicing ophthalmologist. The federal government has embarked on an ambitious program to control payments to physicians in the Medicare program and to reduce the volume of services delivered. It is also attempting to grant more income to physicians engaged in primary care and to those located in rural areas. If national health insurance reform is not adopted, it is likely that many third-party payors will eventually adopt in some fashion the changes instituted by the federal government, because they, too, have a desire to lower cost.

RESOURCE-BASED RELATIVE VALUE SCALE

Congress outlined its plan for changes in the Omnibus Budget Reconciliation Act of 1989. Signed into law in December of that year, it endorsed the concept of a Resource-Based Relative Value Scale (RBRVS) as the basis for future remuneration of physicians. The development of the RBRVS was authorized by Congress in response to suggestions that the current method of payment, based on "usual, customary, and reasonable charges" (UCR), had produced inequity between the amounts paid for procedural services, such as surgery and invasive testing, and evaluation and management ("cognitive") services, such as office visits and hospital care. There was concern that this imbalance might possibly exert undue influence on the frequency with which the more remunerative services were performed, and might also influence medical students to choose future specialty training on the basis of financial considerations. In addition, the current system was felt by many health policy advisors to be inflationary, unduly complex, and not subject to the usual competitive restraints of the marketplace.[117]

Through HCFA, Congress then mandated a study contracted to William Hsiao, PhD, and his associates at the Harvard School of Public Health (the "Hsiao Study"), which authorized the development of an alternative system of reimbursement for physicians based on the cost of the resources expended for provision of health care. The study evaluated the total work performed by the physician in providing each service and subdivided it into component parts of time, mental effort and judgment, technical skill and physical effort, and stress. It also included an analysis of practice costs and attempted to account for loss of income due to added years of specialty training.

As expected, the study demonstrated that current reimbursement levels for the "cognitive services" undervalued them and that many of the procedural services were "overpriced."[118] The Hsiao data indicated a reduction of almost 41% in future income for ophthalmologists under the new system. The methods and conclusions of the study were reassessed by the Physician Payment Review Commission (PPRC), an advisory body created in 1986 by Congress to provide input on Medicare payment reform and to develop a new system of payment. The PPRC modified some of the RBRVS study's assumptions and estimated that the overall decrease for ophthalmology will be closer, on average, to 17%.[119]

In addition to the modifications proposed by the PPRC, there were many deficiencies in the original Hsiao study. These included inadequate estimates of pre- and postservice work, inadequate assessment of subspecialty procedures, and inadequate response rates for many of the procedures studied. For this reason, a second study by Hsiao was commissioned and funded by the American Academy of Ophthalmology and the ASCRS. This study corrected many of the methodologic errors in initial analysis, provided for separate polling of specialists in cornea and retina, and gave a better estimate of the time and work involved in pre- and postoperative care. Although significant problems remained, the results of this effort (Hsiao Phase II) were used to make the final determination of fees under the RBRVS system.

When the initial rules for RBRVS were released by HCFA in June of 1991,[120] they produced a firestorm of criticism. Over 95,000 comments from physicians and other interested parties were received during the review period, resulting in the incorporation of significant changes (generally beneficial to physicians). Initially published in the Federal Register in 1991,[121] the rules have since been modified again by HCFA[122] for 1993. These changes, many of which were also beneficial to physicians, were initiated in many instances by comments from individual physicians, the AMA Relative Value Update Committee (RUC), and the Academy. Some of the highlights are summarized in the sections below.

MEDICARE PHYSICIAN FEE SCHEDULE

Beginning in 1992 and continuing through 1996, there has been a gradual movement towards the Medicare Fee Schedule payment levels (Fig. 2.21). This system determines fees paid to physicians by a complex formula (Fig. 2.22) that takes into account the relative work performed, malpractice costs, and office overhead, all modified by geographic indices that purport to correct for the variance in cost of these factors in various parts of the country. The figure generated is then multiplied by a nationwide conversion factor ($31.001 for both medical and surgical services in 1992, $31.962/$31.249 for surgical/medical in 1993) to arrive at the Medicare Fee Schedule (MFS) amount. Initially, if the payment arrived at by this calculation was within ±15% of the MFS amount, the fee went immediately to the MFS payment. If

---

FIGURE 2.21. Formula for Physician Payment Under Medicare Fee Schedule

$$\text{Payment} = [(RVU_w \times GPCI_w) + (RVU_{oh} \times GPCI_{oh}) + (RVU_m \times GPCI_m)] \times CF$$

where

RVU_w	= physician work relative value units for the service.
RVU_{oh}	= overhead relative value units for the service.
RVU_m	= malpractice relative value units for the service.
$GPCI_w$	= geographic practice cost index value for physician work applicable in the locality.
$GPCI_{oh}$	= geographic practice cost index value for overhead applicable in the locality.
$GPCI_m$	= geographic practice cost index value for malpractice applicable in the locality.
CF	= uniform national conversion factor.

Source: Health Care Financing Administration.

FIGURE 2.22. Implementation Schedule for Medicare Fee Schedule

1992	Payment for services with historical payments within 15% of the fee schedule amount paid at the fee schedule amount.
	Payment for services with historical payments below 85% of the fee schedule amount paid at the historical rate plus 15% of the fee schedule amount.
	Payment for services with historical payments above 115% of the fee schedule amount paid at the historical rate less 15% of the fee schedule amount.
1993	Payment based on 75% of the updated 1992 payment amount and 25% of the fee schedule amount.
1994	Payment based on 67% of the updated 1993 payment amount and 33% of the fee schedule amount.
1995	Payment based on 50% of the updated 1994 payment amount and 50% of the fee schedule amount.
1996	Payment based on the fee schedule.

Adapted from the Physician Payment Review Commission, 1991 Report to Congress.

not, there will be a gradual transition towards the MFS amount until it is reached in 1996. Under the original plan, the MFS value for cataract extraction with lens implant in 1996 (not counting future MFS updates or changes due to volume performance considerations) would be approximately $940. Proposed budgetary reforms introduced by President Clinton could lower that figure to $607.[123]

There are significant changes in the 1993 HCFA reimbursement policies affecting ophthalmology which are beneficial (Fig. 2.23). Retinal laser codes (CPT 67210 and 67228), which were significantly undervalued in 1992 because of changes in the CPT interpretation of the service performed, had significant increases in their work relative value units (RVUs). These increases, which averaged over 50%, were a compromise to take into account that treatments are frequently spread over several sessions to increase both safety and efficacy. Pseudophakic corneal transplant (CPT 65755), which was also grossly undercompensated in 1992, underwent a significant change, with the total RVU almost doubling to 41.45. Only nine codes had a decrease in RVU for work, with Yag capsulotomy (66821) being the most notable. Values for cataract extraction with lens implant (CPT 66984) were unchanged. Significant changes in ophthalmic practice expense and malpractice RVUs for certain procedures occurred as well.[124]

FIGURE 2.23. Relative Work Value Changes, 1993

THESE 10 PROCEDURES HAD THEIR WORK VALUE INCREASED MORE THAN 20% BY HCFA.

CPT #	PROCEDURE	CHANGE
65436	Curette/treat cornea	40%
65820	Relieve inner eye pressure	21%
65850	Incision of eye	32%
66130	Remove eye lesion	95%
66605	Removal of iris	46%
67210	Treatment of retinal lesion	44%
67228	Treatment of retinal lesion	84%
67335	Eye suture during surgery	141%
67345	Destroy nerve of eye muscle	28%
67570	Decompress optic nerve	34%

THE RVU WORK VALUES OF THESE 9 PROCEDURES WERE REDUCED APPROXIMATELY 3% BY HCFA.

CPT #	PROCEDURE
65112	Remove eye, revise socket
65710	Corneal transplant
66821	Lasering secondary cataract
66840	Removal of lens material
67036	Removal of inner eye material
67107	Repair detached retina
67108	Repair detached retina
67141	Treatment of retina
67145	Treatment of retina

Source: Ocular Surgery News, February 1, 1993, p. 39.

Overall, HCFA reviewed values for approximately 800 codes for 1993. Most remained the same, but 10 times as many were raised as lowered. This resulted in an estimate by the HCFA that overall Medicare expenses would increase by $450 million in 1993. Because by statute the HCFA cannot increase fees by anywhere close to that amount, it was decided that *all* procedures would have their total RVU reduced by 2.8%. Unlike the practice expense and professional liability insurance values discussed earlier, geographic practice cost indices were not modified at all, even though many analysts believe that they, too, are not very accurate.[125] HCFA estimates that for 1993 the percent change in allowed charges for ophthalmology will be a decrease of 0.2%.[124]

CONVERSION FACTOR

There remains a great deal of controversy concerning the fairness of the method used to calculate the first conversion factor value. Initially it was proposed to be $26.87, a number chosen to compensate for the assumed increase in the volume and intensity level of physician services that would occur in response to a lowering of fees (the "behavioral offset"). HCFA felt, for a variety of reasons, that the entire increase could be dealt with only by reducing the conversion factor. However, this method would have resulted in a net reduction of payments to physicians of several billion dollars, violating the intent of Congress that the implementation of RBRVS be budget neutral. In addition, because the conversion factor is permanent, its decrease would have had a deleterious effect on reimbursement levels long after the transition period for RBRVS had expired.

After extensive criticism of this method by the AMA and all specialty societies, a compromise was reached. Instead of using only the conversion factor to calculate the fee changes, the transition adjustment was implemented by reducing the historical payment base (the 1991 average Medicare-allowed amount) by 5.5% (see Fig. 2.22). This change, as well as several others of a more technical nature, allowed the conversion factor to be increased to $31.001 for 1992. This figure still contains a behavioral offset component, an assumption most physicians consider to be unfair because there is a separate, specific process (the Medicare Volume Performance Standard—MVPS) that is supposed to compensate for any additional increase in services by reducing payments in subsequent years (see below). For 1993, the conversion factor increased for surgical services by 3.1% (from $31.001 to $31.962), compared with only 0.8% (from $31.001 to $31.249) for medical services. This higher increase for surgical codes was due to the fact that surgeons kept their dollar volume increase for 1992 below predetermined limits, whereas payments for nonsurgical services exceeded them.

MEDICARE VOLUME PERFORMANCE STANDARDS

Although the initial payment reform recommendations were required to be budget neutral, MVPSs were proposed that will link future payments to physicians with the volume of services performed in the preceding year. The MVPS will be the primary mechanism of control of total spending on physician services. Development of this system (which differs very little from the expenditure targets vigorously opposed by organized medicine) was deemed necessary because the amount spent per Medicare beneficiary increased from

$280 in 1978 to $1,072 in 1988 (despite fee freezes and reductions), with the number of services per beneficiary increasing from 12 to 24. Part of this increase was due to the tendency of physicians to increase the frequency and intensity of services rendered as the reimbursement per service decreases.

The MVPS decrees that if the increase in Medicare expenditures for payment for physician services exceeds the amount projected and allowed by Congress, fees during the following fiscal year will be reduced proportionally; if the expenditures are less than projected (most unlikely if the factors that stimulated the development of the MVPS are considered), they will be increased proportionally. The present law requires the HHS to recommend an MVPS based on inflation, changes in technology, size and composition of the Medicare population, and any evidence of inappropriate usage of services. After the Physician Payment Plan Review Commission (PPRC) also makes a recommendation, Congress determines the value for the following fiscal year. If Congress is unable or unwilling to act, there is a default formula that automatically sets the rate. Organized medicine objected to this provision as a form of medical care rationing, but was unsuccessful in defeating it. The MVPSs for surgery and medicine are currently considered separately (Fig. 2.24).

FIGURE 2.24. Volume Performance Standards and Conversion Factor Updates, 1990–1993

		PERCENT INCREASE	
YEAR	**TOTAL**	**SURGICAL**	**NONSURGICAL**
1990			
Final	9.1	...	...
Actual growth	10.6	...	...
1991			
HHC	9.9	8.7	10.5
PPRC	11.2	9.3	12.1
Final	7.3	3.3	8.6
Actual growth	8.6	2.9	10.5
1992			
HHS	6.2	4.1	7.1
PPRC	8.6	6.6	9.6
Final	10.0	6.5	11.2
Actual growth (preliminary)	6.0	-0.6	8.5
1993			
HHS	7.3	6.0	7.9
PPRC	8.9	8.9	8.9
Final	10.0	8.4	10.8

Source: PPRC Report to Congress, 1993, p. 230.

In November of 1992, Congress determined the MVPS for 1993 to be 8.4% for surgery and 10.8% for all nonsurgical services. The maintenance of separate medical and surgical standards for 1993 was opposed by almost every organized medical group except the American College of Surgery. A fierce battle developed because in 1991 (the year that determines spending for fiscal 1993), surgeons remained within their spending limit of a 3.3% increase. Other services increased at a rate of 10.6%, which exceeded the limit of 8.6%. This would therefore have required the latter group to have an allowable fee increase of only 0.3%, whereas surgical payments could jump by 2.6%. Such a policy would be in direct conflict with the goal of RBRVS, which was to increase primary care reimbursement at the expense of surgical income.

The AMA and other groups lobbied in favor of a single MVPS that gave a larger increase to primary care services. However, Congress was reluctant to drop the separate standard that had been promised to the surgical groups as a reward for their backing of RBRVS in 1991. Eventually, HHS and the PPRC (the two groups required by law to advise Congress) both agreed that the separate standards should be maintained for 1993. Congress, following its usual policy of avoiding difficult and controversial decisions whenever possible, chose to let the default formula set the actual values, which resulted in a greater increase than that suggested by the two advisory panels.[126]

Data are now available indicating that the volume increases predicted by HCFA as fees were reduced were too high, resulting in behavioral offsets that reduced reimbursement to physicians by more than the amount needed to preserve budget neutrality (see the discussion above on the conversion factor). The increased volume observed was actually largest in the nonsurgical services, but even for those it was only half of that projected by government agencies. Balance billing also fell by 34%, reducing physician income still further.[127]

Hence, it appears that the net increase in Medicare spending for 1993 will be well below the 10% allowed. This should result in an *increase* in physician fees for fiscal 1994 but is unlikely to do so, since the Clinton administration has shown no interest in increasing physician income or raising Medicare expenses. In fact, it is likely that additional *reductions* in reimbursement will be proposed.[128,129]

PARTICIPATING VERSUS NONPARTICIPATING STATUS

Medicare participation requires that physicians agree to accept the Medicare Fee Schedule amount as payment in full for *all* covered services rendered to *all* Medicare patients for a given period, usually 1 year. In general, nonparticipating physicians do not have to accept assignment on any beneficiary who is not Medicaid eligible but may do so selectively if they wish. They can charge the patient about 9% more than those who participate. This represents a significant reduction over charges allowed in the past, and is consistent with the government's desire to "encourage" more and more physicians to participate.

Noncovered services, such as refraction and elective cosmetic procedures, can be billed directly to the patient whether or not the physician participates. In 1992, over 66% of ophthalmologists chose to be participating physicians,[130] and the number is likely to increase in the future if present trends continue and the amount that can be balance-billed to the patients decreases. A detailed discussion of the pros and cons of participating is contained in Chapter 5.

The rules are particularly onerous for new physicians. They are reimbursed at only 80% of the fee schedule amount in the first year, with an increase of only 5% a year until they reach parity. In addition, the definition proposed for new physicians is quite strict, requiring them to be in practice during the first full 6 months of the calendar year to qualify. Because most new physicians start in July rather than January, this means that many will work for almost 18 months at the first-year new physician rate. Fortunately, this reduction does not apply for the primary care evaluation and management codes and for physicians who practice in specifically designated rural areas.

NEW PHYSICIANS

The global surgery policies under the new system will be different also. For major surgery, the initial office evaluation or consultation will remain billable as a separate charge. All additional preoperative visits by the surgeon, the actual surgical procedure, and 90 days of postoperative care will be contained in the package, including treatment of complications that do not require additional operating room time. Complications requiring repeat surgery will be billable separately but at a reduced rate. Consultations requested from other physicians by the operating surgeon (such as preoperative medical evaluations) will be billable by those physicians.

GLOBAL SURGERY POLICY

For minor surgery [including many of the starred (*) procedures in the CPT codebook] no payment will be routinely allowed for office visits on the day the procedure is performed unless the visit is for an unrelated problem. The postoperative period will be either 0 or 10 days. The major change for ophthalmology for 1993 involves reduction of payment for Yag laser capsulotomy if performed during the global period for cataract surgery. In addition, the period was changed from 10 days to 0 days for removal of superficial external ocular foreign bodies. Each procedure in the CPT book has the global period specified in Addendum B in the *Federal Register* (November 25, 1992).

For ophthalmologists who furnish less than the global fee package by delegating postoperative care to another person, the global fee will be reduced by 20%. At present, the HCFA has instituted a policy that refuses to pay for assistants at cataract surgery, although both the AAO and state ophthalmologic societies are challenging this decision.

Limited-license practitioners (such as optometrists) will be paid at the full fee schedule amount for physicians because there is no longer a specialty differential in the CPT codes. In addition, site-of-service differentials will reduce the fees allowed if procedures usually performed in offices are done in outpatient departments. This will be accomplished by reducing the relative value units for practice expense by 50%. For ophthalmology, these initially included laser iridotomy (but not Yag capsulotomy or laser trabeculoplasty), cryo or laser of retinal breaks, treatment of diabetic retinopathy, and several lid and lacrimal procedures. For 1993, CPT codes 67031, 67105, and 68700 have been removed from the list. The complete list is in Addendum F of the *Federal Register* (November 25, 1991).

The HCFA estimated that the new payment policy would decrease payments per service for ophthalmologists by 11% in 1992 but that overall payments would decrease by only 4%. For 1996, the payments per service will be 21% less than currently, but overall payments will decline by only 11%. It is interesting to note that the budgetary allowance for ophthalmologic services will actually increase by almost 9% annually even with the proposed cuts in

EFFECT ON OPHTHALMOLOGY

reimbursement. The effects on the individual ophthalmologist will depend on the patient mix in the practice. Because office visit reimbursement will increase, some incomes may actually increase, whereas ophthalmologists with high surgical volumes will probably see a decrease. The top 10% of all practices accounts for almost 50% of Medicare-approved charges, and the top 5% for almost 33%. These practices, therefore, will probably bear the brunt of the burden.[131] All practitioners will need to assess carefully their own practice mix to estimate better the effect of the RBRVS on present and future income. Federal health care reform legislation will also greatly influence payments by "traditional" insurance sources (almost certainly decreasing them) and this, too, will have a significant impact on practice income.

Where will all this ultimately lead? According to a *Medical Economics* survey in 1992,[132] ophthalmologists in 1991 ranked eighth (down from third in 1990) in practice income for surgical specialists, with median net practice earnings of $180,280. This dropped ophthalmology below the median income for all surgical specialties for the first time in many years. Remarkably, ophthalmology was the only specialty to show an actual drop in earnings compared with 1989 (Fig. 2.25).

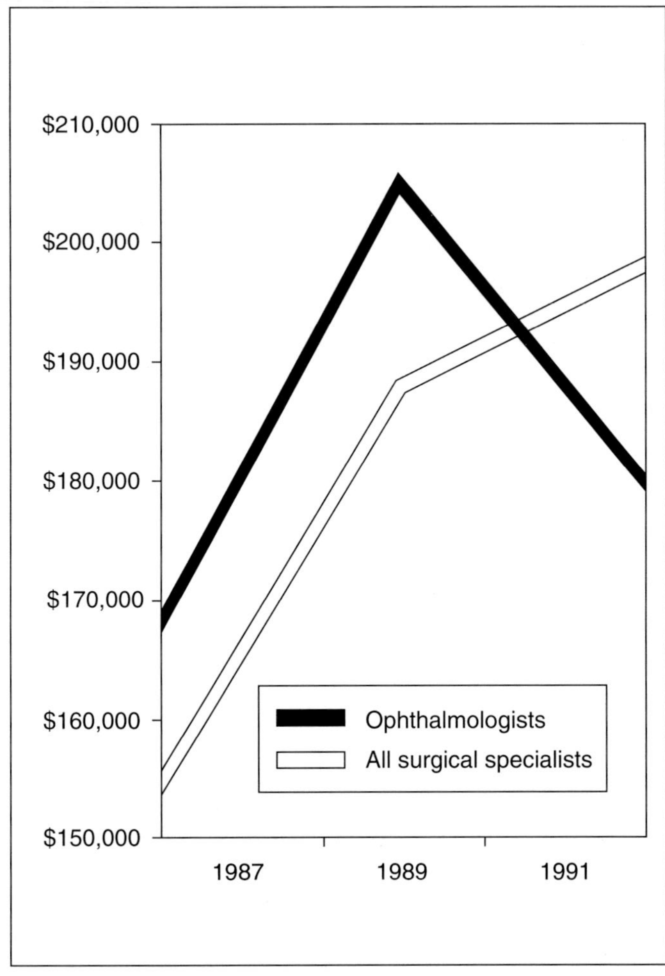

2.25 | Median income: ophthalmologists vs. all surgical specialists. (*Source: Medical Economics,* Apr 12, 1993, p. 90.)

The Physician's Advisor, a respected practice management advisory newsletter, reported that a survey of the Society of Medical–Dental Consultants' members' clients indicated that dispensing ophthalmologists reported gross profit (income left after paying all expenses except physician salary and benefits) of $354,500 with 55% overhead, with nondispensing practitioners reporting gross profit of $279,000 and overhead of 47.9%.[133] These physicians represent the upper echelon of practices in terms of sophistication and financial success (as shown by the fact that they can afford a consultant!), and usually show gross profits above the median.

Despite the problems that loom large, it is clear that, in addition to the intellectual challenge and satisfaction inherent in an ophthalmologic career, it remains a wonderful way to earn a living. It is likely to remain so in the future, although in a much more complicated and competitive environment.

RISK MANAGEMENT AND MALPRACTICE

Over the last 20 years there has been rising concern within the medical community regarding the crisis in medical malpractice litigation. Growing numbers of claims, coupled with large awards, have caused the cost of malpractice insurance to rise at an alarming pace. Between 1974 and 1978 malpractice insurance was simply unavailable in many parts of the country, as commercial insurers withdrew in response to substantial losses. This situation led to the development of many of the physician-owned, not-for-profit companies that write a significant number of the malpractice policies in force today.

In the mid-1980s, the most recent phase of the crisis, malpractice insurance remained available but premiums sometimes doubled within a year and grew at an overall average annual rate of 21.9%. This made them the fastest rising component of overhead for physicians in practice.[1] More recently, in response to a decrease in the number of claims being filed, premium rates seem to have stabilized and, in some cases, have actually fallen slightly.[2] It is hoped that this trend will continue.

The threat of malpractice litigation has a direct negative impact on the availability of medical care. Rising liability costs for obstetricians have added over $1,000 to the cost of a routine delivery in Florida. Nationwide, many obstetricians have simply stopped providing obstetric services, particularly for high-risk patients. Family practitioners have done the same thing, leaving many states with entire counties that lack these vital services.

Liability costs also increase the cost of medical care directly by increasing the prevalence of "defensive medicine"—tests and procedures performed with the primary intent of avoiding liability risk. These tests alone added an estimated $11.7 billion to the cost of medical care in 1985. As noted by former Health and Human Services Secretary Dr. Otis Bowen, "A child falls off a swing and bumps his head. In the old days, you'd tell him to go home and put ice on it. Now you give him $100 worth of x-rays and maybe a CAT scan, and *then* (emphasis added) you tell him to go home and put ice on it."[3]

The crisis in liability litigation extends outside of medicine as well. In 1988, injury cases cost United States railroads 43% of their profits, with awards of $880 million dollars.[4]

Research and development of new products in the medical field are stifled by concern for potential product liability problems, and even products that are state of the art in terms of safety are not immune to challenge. Imposition of punitive damages, often many times greater than the compensatory award involved, is also becoming more common. According to a poll of chief executives of large American companies, the costs of dealing with these problems contribute significantly to the difficulty of United States industry in competing with products from abroad.[5]

Unlike the present situation in medical malpractice litigation, in which the number of large jury awards appears to be decreasing, the number of large verdicts in nonmedical cases continues to climb. In 1989, $547 million was awarded to individuals in the 10 largest cases, with the highest single amount ($76 million) awarded for shipyard asbestos exposure.[6]

THE GENERAL PROBLEM OF MEDICAL MALPRACTICE

How widespread is the problem of medical malpractice? Although hard data are difficult to come by, a recent review of hospital care in New York State by researchers from the Harvard School of Public Health indicates that 1.3% of 30,000 patients studied had a "negligent adverse event" during their stay. Ironically, only 47 of the patients studied filed malpractice claims, and 39 of those were filed in cases where researchers found no evidence of negligence.[7] This corroborates previous studies indicating that only one of ten potentially legitimate malpractice claims reaches the court system.

When cases do reach the courts, they are handled under the system of tort law, a civil proceeding that involves payments to persons for a wrongful act committed against them. This system is intended to provide compensation to an injured party, as well as to ensure professional accountability and, in theory, to serve also as a deterrent to any further improper activities. There is concern, however, that a doctrine of strict liability, in which the physician is held liable for a bad outcome regardless of who is at fault, is increasingly being applied by juries sympathetic to a plaintiff who has suffered obvious impairment of function.

There is also a growing body of evidence to suggest that the present system may not be the most efficient way of handling cases. Studies by the RAND Corporation indicate that more than 50% of insurance company malpractice premium income is spent on claim resolution rather than on patient compensation. A significant portion of this money is spent on claims ultimately decided in favor of the defendant physician, in which the patient receives no compensation whatsoever.[1] Even in cases that do come to trial, almost 70% are decided in favor of the defendant physician.

Although the present contingency fee system is defended by those who believe that it is the only way to provide access to the courts for those of limited means, it is obvious that this premise holds true only for situations in which the potential judgment will be large enough to cover the costs of preparing the case. Cases involving small sums, and those particularly difficult to present, may never be accepted by attorneys, even when a legal basis for malpractice is evident.

THE EXPERIENCE OF OPHTHALMOLOGY

It is useful for ophthalmologists to look specifically at their own experience rather than at the overall malpractice situation. In general, the same risk factors that apply to all physicians also apply to ophthalmologists. Better-informed patients, heightened expectations, dissatisfaction with the manner of treatment by physician and/or staff, charge and office procedure complaints, and less than optimal results all increase the chance of a malpractice complaint being filed. Conversely, a kind, compassionate, and attentive physician who runs a caring office and takes time to talk with and explain things to patients may avoid having a malpractice suit filed even if a poor outcome occurs.

A review by the General Accounting Office of malpractice claims closed in 1984 revealed that ophthalmologists were responsible for only 3% of the claims filed nationwide. Fifteen percent of ophthalmologists in practice at the time were involved in these claims, of which only one third settled with some form of payment to the plaintiff.[8]

In Louisiana, a review panel that evaluates potential medical malpractice claims has been active since 1975. Between 1978 and 1986, 99 complaints were filed against ophthalmologists, representing about 2% of all malpractice claims presented to the panel. Ninety percent of the cases were decided in favor of the ophthalmologists, and in only three cases was the ruling against them. Since 1977, only 11 cases have been settled against ophthalmologists in Louisiana, with just one for damages in excess of $100,000. The largest award was for a perforated globe; the other claims dealt primarily with cataract surgery.[9]

A recently published retrospective review of a large series of nonrandomly selected medicolegal claims against ophthalmologists showed that, of 700 cases, most did not even go to trial. Of those that did come to trial, over half were decided in favor of the ophthalmologist. Lack of good rapport between patient and physician was an important risk factor in the instigation of many of the claims.[10]

The American Academy of Ophthalmology also has a malpractice insurance program designed for its members. Ophthalmic Mutual Insurance Company (OMIC), founded in October of 1987, revealed to policy holders that it had processed a total of 371 claims as of March 1992, of which 240 had been closed without payment to the plaintiff. One hundred seven remained open, and only 24 had required settlement with payment. Half of the claims filed involved cataract surgery (Fig. 3.1). There were four cases of endophthalmitis, and six cases were concerned with implantation of lenses of incorrect power. Ten percent of the claims involved retinal detachment surgery and a similar percentage dealt with failure to diagnose. The largest payment was for failure to diagnose a lung tumor present on a preoperative chest x-ray, and no settlement for a case more directly related to ophthalmology was in excess of $100,000.[11]

Figure 3.1. Percentage of Ophthalmology Claims by Service, 1992

PROCEDURE OR SERVICE	% (N=371)
Cataract	44%
Retina/Vitreous	18%
Glaucoma	4%
Medical	7%
Radial keratotomy	1%
All others	26%

Source: OMIC, Claims Analysis, October 1987–March 1992.

DEFINITION OF MALPRACTICE

In general, to prove a medical malpractice action, a patient must establish that:

1. The physician had a duty of care to the patient
2. There was an act or omission by the physician that failed to meet the requisite standard of care
3. The act or omission was negligently performed
4. The injury experienced by the patient was causally connected to the act or omission in question

The proof of a malpractice action further depends on demonstrating a deviation from the ordinary standard of care that would have been given under similar circumstances by other members of the medical profession.[12] The mere occurrence of an adverse result does not constitute presumptive evidence of malpractice. In most instances, adequate proof that the actions involved did deviate from accepted standards requires the use of an expert witness, unless the personal testimony of the physician or the act itself clearly indicates that the standard has not been met *(res ipsa loquitor)*.

In most states it is also possible to assign a portion of the fault to the plaintiff. This can occur, for example, if it can be documented that the plaintiff failed to follow instructions or to return for scheduled visits. In addition, patients are expected to exercise reasonable effort to seek medical care if indicated to avoid further injury, even if the injury itself stems from negligent medical care.[13]

DAMAGES

Compensatory medical malpractice awards are usually divided into several portions, i.e., general damages and special damages. General damages consist of pain and suffering, whereas special damages are concerned with lost wages and with actual and potential medical expenses. In addition, punitive damages, a penalty specifically designed as a deterrent to other similar actions, can also be awarded.[14] This additional remuneration, the size of which can be many times the actual compensatory award, is usually not covered by malpractice insurance.

TORT REFORM

Because of the many difficulties discussed above, pressure has been exerted to modify the system presently in place to compensate those injured by negligent medical practice. These efforts, generally grouped under the title of tort reform, are being pursued at both the state and federal levels (Fig. 3.2). The initial impetus for these efforts was the malpractice insurance crisis in the mid-1970s and 1980s, but continuing problems have resulted in a steady flow of additional suggestions intended to help stem the tide.

Figure 3.2. Key Elements in Tort Reform

Elimination of joint and several liability
Review panels
Sliding scale limits on contingency fees
Structured payouts of future awards
Limits on noneconomic damages
No-fault malpractice insurance
Mandatory offset of collateral payments

Modification or elimination of joint and several liability provisions has been a major focus of tort reform efforts. This concept requires the owner of the "deepest pocket" available to pay the judgment or a major component of it, even if the primary responsibility for the negligence was not his own. Although it has not been possible in most instances to do away with the doctrine entirely, modifications have been made in many jurisdictions to lessen its impact on physicians. One of these requires juries to apportion the degree of fault attributable to each party in the suit (including those who may have previously been released from liability) and holds defendants responsible only for their own individual portion. Another modification declares that defendants are obligated to share joint and several liability only with other defendants whose proportional share of the fault is equal to or less than their own.

Establishment of review panels or procedures to evaluate claims before they are filed is also being tried in many states. The intent of these panels is to reduce the number of nuisance actions by deciding before the court becomes involved whether or not there is a reasonable cause of action. Some panels require sworn testimony from a health care provider indicating that the defendant deviated from the customary standard of care and that the patient suffered as a result.

Sliding scale limits on contingency fee percentages for plaintiffs' attorneys have also been proposed and in some cases instituted. These provide for significant decreases in the percentage paid to the attorney as the size of the award increases. This policy is intended to encourage attorneys to be more willing to accept cases involving smaller amounts of money and also to promote more out-of-court settlements for reasonable sums, since the financial incentive for the attorney to press for a particularly large settlement is reduced.

Along the same lines, limits on noneconomic damages have been proposed. These, which include pain and suffering, loss of enjoyment of life, and other factors difficult for juries to assess in economic terms, are often a major portion of the large settlements that have been obtained.

Periodic payout of future awards lessens the immediate financial burden for insurance companies (the judgments can be funded by annuity or other similar arrangements). It also ensures that the money will actually be available in the future for the injured patient, and will not be misappropriated or otherwise misspent. It also provides for ending the future medical payments portion of the judgment if death occurs. This reduces the cost to the insurance company and, it is hoped, malpractice premium costs as well.

Often patients have several types of insurance coverage that may also reimburse them for expenses and/or wages lost as a result of accident or injury. Mandatory offset of collateral sources of payment is an important provision that makes the malpractice judgment net of all other sources of compensation, avoiding the problem of double payment of medical expenses and lost wages.

Institution of compensation for certain losses regardless of who was at fault (so-called no-fault malpractice insurance) provides another way of reducing malpractice costs. It allows the payments to be made without the expense of determining individual culpability. This plan could lead to compensation of victims of malpractice more fairly, because all injured patients would have access to the system. Although it would probably reduce the number of very large awards and might possibly decrease medical costs overall by decreasing litigation expenses and the waste of "defensive medicine," overall costs could increase because access to the system would be easier. Similar systems are presently in place for settling Workers' Compensation cases at the state level and, under federal law, for vaccine injuries.

GOVERNMENTAL EFFORTS ON TORT REFORM
STATE MEASURES

Attempts to institute tort reforms have been, in general, most successful at the state level.[1] In California, for example, the Medical Injury Compensation Recovery Act incorporated many of the suggestions in the proposal discussed previously. This act, declared constitutional in 1985, saved the physician-owned malpractice carriers in the state $6.5 million in 1987 alone. It also had the apparent effect of promoting more out-of-court settlements of meritorious cases for more reasonable sums, and cut the time from occurrence of an incident to closing of a claim by 1 year.

Another state statute, that of Virginia which places a ceiling on the award for all damages in a malpractice action, has been held constitutional by both the Virginia State Supreme Court and the Fourth United States Circuit Court of Appeals. This is the first case in which a ceiling on total damages in a medical malpractice has been upheld at the federal level. Several other state courts have upheld limitations on noneconomic damages, but others have declared them unconstitutional, and further challenges at both the federal and state levels are likely.

FEDERAL MEASURES

At the federal level, a 1987 Department of HHS Liability Task Force recommended that extensive tort reform be instituted to help control the medical malpractice liability crisis. Several bills were also introduced in Congress in 1990,[15] one of which (the Lawsuit Reform Act) would create federal statutes that would apply in all tort cases. The provisions of this act include:

1. Elimination of joint and several liability
2. Requirement for attorneys to inform clients of available alternatives to litigation
3. Prohibition of damages if the patient's intoxication was in significant part responsible for the injury incurred

Other bills have also been introduced that would place a limit on noneconomic damages, limit attorney's fees, and allow structured settlements of damages in excess of $100,000 (Orin Hatch, S489, 1991). Although progress on these bills has been negligible to date, the fact that they were introduced at all in a body dominated by attorneys indicates an increasing concern about this problem at the federal level. In addition, former President Bush specifically endorsed the concept of tort reform as being an important component of the federal attempt to reduce health care costs.[16]

The AMA has also supported a package of tort reform programs that includes the following provisions:[15]

1. Maximal limit of $250,000 on recovery of noneconomic damages
2. Mandatory offset of collateral sources of patient compensation
3. Sliding scale reduction of attorney contingency fees
4. Periodic payment of awards for future expenses
5. Restriction of the suspension of statute of limitations for minors to 6 years

It is likely that the trial lawyers will actively oppose these federally mandated changes just as they did with similar provisions at the state level.

It is also apparent that the profession itself could do more to evaluate variability in medical care patterns and perhaps lessen the incidence of both iatrogenic injury and medical malpractice. Peer review, based on an educational rather than a punitive approach, can assist in modifying the behavior of physicians whose actions deviate from commonly accepted norms. Actual sanctions should be necessary only in the small number of instances in which repeated departures from acceptable behavior occur after adequate attempts at education and multiple warnings.

It is also likely that an enhanced ability of the medical profession to police itself and to sanction physicians whose treatment consistently falls below acceptable standards will lead to a decrease in malpractice. A number of instances have been documented in which physicians disciplined in one state simply travel to another and continue the practice of medicine. State medical licensure boards often do not adequately investigate credentials presented to them and fail to detect practitioners who are consistently negligent. For this reason, Congress has established the National Practitioner Data Bank as a means of tracking disciplinary actions against individual physicians. This national registry provides hospitals, licensing agencies, and other relevant heath care institutions with information on past professional misconduct, including medical malpractice claim payments, adverse actions on clinical hospital privileges, licensure actions, and society membership actions. Resident physicians are included as well, with the only difference being that clinical privilege actions are exempt from the reporting requirements.[17] All hospitals are required to solicit information from the data bank each time a physician applies for staff privileges and at 2-year intervals for as long as these privileges are maintained. At the present time all medical malpractice payments must be reported, including small sums paid to settle nuisance claims. Unfortunately, this provision will discourage physicians and carriers from settling frivolous claims and will further increase medical malpractice defense costs (and liability insurance premiums). Attempts are being made to exclude small payments from the reporting requirements, but thus far they have been unsuccessful.

The information contained in a physician's file is presently not available to consumer groups or the general public. Each time a report is filed the physician is notified. In addition, physicians have the right to request a copy of their records and to challenge the accuracy of the material presented. The information in dispute will be so marked in the file, but it will not be changed, and it is up to the physician to resolve the dispute with the agency that submitted the original material. In the event that the physician's contentions are supported, every recipient of the original material is supposed to be notified of the change.[18]

The material in the Data Bank is not subject to access under the Freedom of Information Act but, despite the number of safeguards in place, there is still concern that the system can be abused at the expense of innocent physicians. It is hoped, however, that it will, on balance, be helpful in reducing the frequency of repeat malpractice by chronic offenders.

Risk management, a technique devised to assist physicians in understanding and developing ways to prevent malpractice suits, has recently increased in importance. It differs from peer review in that it is less concerned with the actual practice of medicine than with developing methods that document, in

PEER REVIEW

NATIONAL PRACTITIONER DATA BANK

RISK MANAGEMENT

clear, concise, and legible fashion, what was done and why. Failure to support adequately important portions of the medical treatment plan often leads to malpractice actions against physicians who, in truth, were not really guilty of malpractice. Accurate documentation of telephone advice given by the physician or office staff, notification and followup of patients who fail to return for additional care, and documentation of noncompliance with treatment plans are some examples of risk management techniques that protect physicians and at the same time benefit the patient. Specific suggestions for risk management in the ophthalmologist's office are discussed below.

PREFERRED PRACTICE PATTERNS

Development of protocols or guidelines for medical practice can also be useful both for educating physicians and for explaining appropriate treatment parameters to nonphysicians, such as lawyers and juries. Many physicians object to such documents because they feel that they can be used to bolster malpractice claims against them. The AMA has addressed this topic in a recent publication,[12] with the following conclusion:

"Parameters do not create any new liabilities for physicians or payors, nor should parameters increase exposure to already existing liabilities. Proper use of parameters may help physicians and payors better control their existing liability risks.... Physicians need not be concerned that they will be automatically liable for malpractice if they choose to deviate from a practice parameter for legitimate medical reasons and a bad outcome occurs."

The American Academy of Ophthalmology has developed such protocols (called Preferred Practice Patterns, or PPPs) for common ophthalmologic conditions. Although individual ophthalmologists may disagree with portions of the recommendations in these publications, overall they provide a useful framework to assist in the management of frequently encountered ophthalmologic disorders. The PPPs clearly state that they are not meant to be taken in absolute terms by physicians, patients, or others, and that they provide leeway for adjusting the treatment to the specific needs of the individual patient. Copies of the PPPs are available through the Academy.

More recently, a clinical practice guideline dealing with functional visual impairment in adults secondary to cataracts was released by the Agency for Health Care Policy and Research (AHCPR).[19] These guidelines are designed to be used by physicians, nurses, educators, patients, and many other practitioners to help define how cataracts can most effectively be prevented, diagnosed, and treated. The document, written by a multidisciplinary panel that included both academic and practicing ophthalmologists as well as many other health professionals and consumer representatives, deals with the proper approach to and management of visually significant cataracts. Separate versions were created for patients and clinicians, and a detailed literature review is incorporated into the report. The guideline has been endorsed in principle by the American Academy of Ophthalmology, but not by several other large ophthalmologic organizations. Several of them, unhappy with some of the more controversial provisions contained in the document, have created their own version, *Guidelines for Cataract Practice*, which approaches the problem from a slightly different point of view.[20] It is expected that all of these documents will evolve in the future as new information, techniques, and materials become available.

Interest in outcome analysis is also continuing to increase. The ability to specify the range of appropriate outcomes for a given procedure or treatment plan will assist in differentiating between substandard care and a bad result without negligent conduct. Outcome analysis can also assess the efficacy of various treatment methods, making it an excellent educational tool as well. Ophthalmology, with the obvious parameters of preoperative versus postoperative visual acuity for the evaluation of cataract surgery, seems a likely specialty to begin to develop these types of objective treatment assessments.

OUTCOME ANALYSIS

Malpractice insurance compensates patients injured through acts of medical negligence. It is a necessary part of each physician's insurance portfolio, since personal assets are otherwise at risk in the event of an adverse judgment. Various other alternatives, such as "going bare," family trusts, and keeping assets in the name of the spouse or other family members are fraught with hazard (you may be more likely to get divorced than sued for malpractice) and should be avoided. The cost of adequate malpractice insurance for most ophthalmologists is not out of reach (rarely more than 3% to 5% of gross income) and is worth the investment in terms of peace of mind.

MALPRACTICE INSURANCE

In recent years, insurance companies owned by physicians have emerged to provide coverage for medical malpractice. Able to provide adequate coverage at reasonable rates, these companies have the advantage of not having to satisfy the profit needs of outside stockholders, and tend to defend aggressively cases they feel are without merit. Most also have a "consent clause" requiring written permission from the defendant physician before a case can be settled. Many offer a "claims-free discount" to physicians with a favorable claims record. In addition, insureds with an unfavorable claims record or with a pattern of deviation from expected standards of care can be surcharged or prevented from renewing.

The quality and stability of the insurance company are of uppermost importance, because your own assets become the backup if a judgment is rendered against you and your insurer is unable to pay. In recent years, new companies have emerged that are undercapitalized and offer unreasonably low premiums in an effort to attract physicians. You must be certain that the company with which you deal is legitimate. Checking ratings with Best's or other reliable insurance rating services is one way to evaluate the soundness of the company in question.

The structure of the insurance company is also important. Mutual companies have the ability to charge all of their insured physicians an assessment equal to the difference between premium income collected and monies spent to pay claims. In past years these assessments often amounted to several times the initial premium paid. Some mutual companies reinsure risk (contract with other companies to share risk for particularly large claims) so that the actual chance of being assessed is lessened.

Risk retention groups (such as the one sponsored by the AAO) are a special form of insurance company in which some exposure is retained in-house but most of the risk is reinsured with outside groups, such as Lloyd's of London. OMIC, the Academy-sponsored insurance underwriter, is a company of this type, currently retaining $250,000 per claim. This amount then becomes the risk retained by the insured in the event that the company is unable to pay damages because of insolvency. The remainder would be paid by the reinsurer. Fortunately, OMIC is in excellent financial condition, making such a default highly unlikely.

TYPES OF MALPRACTICE INSURANCE

Because of the increasing complexity of medical malpractice policies, it is important for all physicians to read and understand exactly what is covered. Often policies restrict protection for new or controversial procedures without making these exceptions particularly clear. Procedures seldom performed by ophthalmologists are sometimes excluded as well.

Physicians also have certain responsibilities under the policy regarding notification of the company in the event of a potential action against them; failure to follow these procedures properly can result in loss of coverage. The policy also outlines the responsibility of the insurer in the event that a claim is filed, and whether or not the insurer can settle a case without the consent of the insured.

Each type of policy also has specific limits on periods covered and on compensation limits for each event and in the aggregate. Rules vary for continuing protection in the event of voluntary or involuntary retirement, disability, part-time practice, and other situations that may arise. Being familiar with all of this information from the beginning may greatly simplify matters if a crisis occurs.

It is important to understand that a significant time lag usually occurs between the performance of a service that may result in a malpractice action and the date the claim is filed. Only 30% of claims are reported in the year in which the service was actually rendered. By the second year the number increases to 60%, and by the fifth year almost all have been reported.[21]

OCCURRENCE POLICIES

Occurrence policies protect physicians against all claims that *occur* while the policy is in effect, regardless of when the claim is filed. The premium is fixed and no additional assessment can ever be charged for that policy period. Each policy year is unique, and coverage may be changed in future years. The premium structure is level (in contrast to claims-made insurance, in which there are scheduled increases), changing primarily in response to the overall malpractice climate. In general, most ophthalmology training programs provide this type of coverage for residents and fellows.

Because no tail coverage is required (see below), it is possible to switch carriers if there are specific reasons for doing so (e.g., lower premium, better service) without jeopardizing previous coverage. Because the policy is renewed yearly, a fresh aggregate limit for all claims occurring during the policy period is established (i.e., the aggregate limit accumulates), significantly increasing the overall protection available.

CLAIMS-MADE COVERAGE

Claims-made insurance is the most common type of malpractice insurance available today. It was developed because insurance companies became unwilling to extend occurrence protection after having had disastrous experiences with this type of policy in product liability cases such as asbestosis. In that instance, companies found themselves responsible for events that had occurred years earlier when the true risk of the product was unknown and therefore not incorporated into the premium structure in place at the time.

Claims-made malpractice insurance resembles term life insurance in many ways. It provides protection for current exposure only, placing responsibility for obtaining future coverage on the insured. It does this by restricting coverage to events that *occur* and for which a claim *is filed* during the policy period. Because the number of claims filed during the first few years is small, the premium is initially low and then gradually increases over 3 to 5 years to a "mature rate," which is usually relatively stable and is similar to the premium charged for occurrence policies.

However, when a claims-made policy is terminated, protection must be obtained against adverse events that may have occurred but have not yet been reported. This "extended reporting endorsement" (commonly referred to as a tail) may cost from 50% to 200% of the last premium paid, based on the past insurance history and the number of years the claims-made policy has been in effect.

Because the cost of the tail is quite variable, it is difficult to calculate the total cost of the insurance coverage until after the tail is purchased. This makes comparison of different policies difficult. It also makes it difficult to switch companies, since a tail must either be purchased from the current company or from the new company (if available) as retroactive coverage (this is often called a nose). This situation may leave the insured physician in the position of having to deal with two separate underwriting entities.

Recently there has been developed a free-standing tail policy that is portable and can be purchased over several years while the physician is still in practice.[22] This allows the premiums to be tax deductible (unlike those paid after retirement), and the policy travels with the physician if there is a change in insurance carrier.

Unlike occurrence policies, claims-made policies have no aggregate limit accumulation. Therefore, the dollar limit of the tail purchased usually represents the total amount available to cover all claims filed in the future. It must therefore be high enough to account for future inflation. On the other hand, increased protection against future claims can sometimes be purchased (i.e., the tail coverage can be larger than the coverage prevailing during the regular policy years), a benefit not available for occurrence policies.

CLAIMS-PAID INSURANCE

This type of coverage protects only against claims that *occur, are filed,* and *are paid* during the policy period. Because of the usual lag between the moment an event occurs and the time payment takes place, the initial premiums for this type of insurance are not very high. However, to retain protection, the insured becomes, in effect, locked in with the company, because switching companies once a claim has been filed but not paid is quite difficult. This type of policy should be approached with great caution, since adverse judg-

Figure 3.3 Malpractice Insurance Types and Payment Policy

	EVENTS NEEDED WITHIN POLICY PERIOD TO ENSURE PAYMENT		
TYPE OF INSURANCE	INCIDENT	CLAIM	PAYMENT
Occurrence	Yes	No	No
Claims made	Yes	Yes	No
Claims paid	Yes	Yes	Yes

ments not protected by adequate reinsurance can result in a significant assessment and/or premium increase. Moreover, as additional assessments occur, physicians who have no claims pending against them may leave the company to avoid the higher cost. This leaves behind those who do have claims pending, since they have nowhere else to turn. As the number of insured physicians decreases, the price to those remaining (on a per capita basis) increases, and the initial low premium outlay may be eclipsed by this additional expense.

Some features of each type of policy are outlined in Figure 3.3.

RISK MANAGEMENT IN THE OPHTHALMOLOGIST'S OFFICE

Malpractice suits are filed for many reasons, not all of which relate directly to inadequate or substandard medical care. As mentioned previously, in some instances when actual malpractice may have occurred, and in many cases with bad results, no claim is ever filed. Under similar circumstances, other physicians may find themselves not so lucky. Some of the factors that may determine into which group you fall are discussed below. Many of these suggestions were adapted from *The Risk Controller,* a newsletter circulated by Risk Control Associates, Inc., a Missouri physician-owned medical liability insurer. The AMA[23] and the AAO[24] have also recently published risk management guidelines for office personnel.

GOOD PATIENT RELATIONS

It has been said that patients rarely sue physicians they like, even in the face of less than optimal results. In general, that statement holds true. Many patients sue because they are angry and feel that legal action is the only way to get back at the doctor. Therefore, it is incumbent on all physicians to pay particular attention to policies and procedures, for themselves and their office staff, that encourage patient loyalty and good relations.

Taking the time to get to know patients and to establish good rapport is the most helpful technique of all. Medicine has traditionally been a personal services profession, in which the degree of patient comfort with a given physician is often more important than the years of specialty training, rank in medical school, and other objective criteria. Practices grow and prosper because of referrals from satisfied patients.

Development of the skills needed to foster successful relationships—the "art of medicine"—is not something easily taught. Although not every physician is comfortable in dealing with individuals on an intimate and personal level, it is possible for almost everyone to be kind, considerate, and to seem interested in patients as people, not just as disease entities. For most patients, that will do quite nicely.

Patients also get upset with physicians for a variety of reasons, not all of which are justified. In general, long waits for appointments and while in the office constitute the most frequent patient complaint. Depersonalization of medical care, high fees and preoccupation with making money, rude staff and ancillary personnel, and inadequate time spent with patients are also commonly mentioned.

Failure to provide enough information to enable the patient to participate intelligently in treatment decisions may also promote discontent. Inattention to requests to provide information for insurance companies and employers can cost patients money and make them angry. Exerting special efforts to prevent these types of problems is time well spent.

What is the best way to handle patients with complaints? In general, the physician should personally discuss the problem with the patient. Most of the time, delegation of this responsibility to the staff only adds to the problem. The complaint should be discussed in a calm and professional manner, without necessarily admitting fault. Do not make promises that you cannot fulfill. Remember that a patient's medical history cannot be discussed with any outside party without written permission from the patient.

Frequently, complaints deal with fees. Many times the simplest way to handle the situation is to adjust the fee accordingly. Doing so is not an admission of fault or guilt, or that the original charge was excessive. The time saved and the patient goodwill engendered are often worth the small cost involved. Only the physician should make this decision, although a general office policy should be in place for handling this type of problem.

INFORMED CONSENT

Patient consent must be obtained before medical or surgical procedures are instituted. Obtaining "informed consent" is considered a required standard of medical care today. It is important because the patient has the right to be an active participant in deciding whether or not to undergo a given treatment or procedure and cannot do so without having all of the pertinent information available. Simply signing a consent form is not the same as giving informed consent.

It is clear that informed consent implies an understanding of the procedure or treatment in question. Not only must the explanation be understandable in layman's terms, but all questions must be satisfactorily answered in a way that patients can clearly comprehend. For practices with a significant number of patients for whom English is not the primary language, consideration should be given to having explanatory materials and consent forms printed in the appropriate language. Bilingual staff may also be essential if the physician does not possess that skill.

For a patient to win a judgment regarding physician failure to obtain informed consent, it is necessary to prove that the patient was not given the information necessary to make the proper decision, and to prove that if such information had been provided another course of action would have been chosen. The plaintiff must also show that there was an injury as a result of the treatment that was chosen and that the injury was related to undisclosed risks.

The physician should inform the patient. Nonphysicians can assist in education and communication with the patient, but it is ultimately the responsibility of the physician to be certain that the information provided before treatment is adequate. When practical, the consent should be obtained well in advance of the procedure.

In most situations, documentation of informed consent should be in writing and the patient should sign the consent form in the presence of a witness. In signing, the witness simply indicates that the signature of the patient was not forced. It is often helpful to have one or more family members present. Jargon and technical terms should be avoided. Oral consent is also binding, but is more difficult to document, making it easier for the patient to deny later. In the rare instance in which the patient waives the right to be informed, documentation of this in the record is of utmost importance.

The first step in obtaining informed consent is to tell the patient the diagnosis(es) if known, or the differential diagnosis if the situation is less clear. When possible, the diagnosis should be explained in nonmedical terms. The proposed treatment plan should then be outlined, again as much as possible in layman's terms. The goals of the treatment plan should be explained carefully. The probability of success can be estimated if data are available, but no guarantee should be given that a perfect result will be achieved. Alternative forms of treatment should be presented and similarly discussed, and the prognosis if no treatment is undertaken should be included as well.

The inherent risks of the treatment plan must be explained carefully, especially in situations involving surgery and anesthesia. Although it is difficult to define precisely what must be covered, it should include the information that the "reasonable physician" would provide for the "average patient" to assist in making an "informed decision." Included should be the risk of death or serious disability from anesthesia, significant common complications of the procedure itself, and possible difficulties that can develop during the post-treatment recovery period. All patient questions should be answered, and the fact that this opportunity was offered included in the record.

In addition, if the patient is not legally competent to sign the consent document (e.g., minor children, mentally handicapped adults), be certain that the person who does sign has the proper legal authority to represent the patient. Family members who happen to be immediately available may not be those legally permitted to give consent. In the case of minors, if possible, have the informed consent discussion with both parents and have both sign the form.

Many physicians today make use of commercially prepared videotapes to assist in obtaining informed consent. These tapes explain frequently performed procedures and answer many of the questions patients commonly ask. If such aids are used, they should be previewed by the physician to ensure that the information they present is factually accurate and properly balanced. However, they should never serve as a substitute for the patient–physician dialogue that is always an essential part of obtaining informed consent.

MEDICAL RECORDS

The ultimate defense in any medical malpractice action hinges almost entirely on the medical record. It should be kept current and should accurately and completely document what was done and why. It must detail the patient's complaint, the examination performed to evaluate it, and must provide a summary of the treatment given and the rationale for it. It should also document what was told to the patient and that the patient was given the opportunity to ask whatever questions were felt necessary. All notations should be made in ink or typed to facilitate detection of revisions.

The written document is the only record of events that can be used to defend past actions. Memory of things told to the patient but not recorded may be of little use, so it is wise in every instance to follow the dictum, "if it isn't written, it didn't happen." In addition, records should never be left unattended in the presence of the patient (to avoid tampering) and the patient should never be given the original copy of the record to carry outside the office.

Medical records are legal documents to which patients ultimately have total access. Gratuitous remarks and editorial comments about the patient or family members have no place in it and are to be scrupulously avoided. Similarly, if included at all, comments about former physicians and previous care received should be carefully considered before entry, and the information should be of a factual nature and clearly documented. Otherwise, action for libel may be a risk if the record is produced as part of a legal proceeding.

It is particularly important that all adverse events be completely and carefully documented. Not writing them down does not make them disappear, and their omission may make the explanation of a circumstance much more difficult. The information regarding the event should be detailed (including the treatment instituted and the reason(s) for it), and the results of the intervention must be carefully noted. In addition, what the patient was told about the situation and the patient response should be contained in the record.

It is also important that handwritten records be legible. Typewritten or dictated notes should be signed after proper review by the physician, and all corrections should be initialed and dated. If changes must be made in the record, they should be done in a way that does not obliterate the original entry.

Patient confidentiality considerations must also be carefully observed. Laws for release of information from the medical record vary, but violations can lead to possible civil or criminal action against the physician. Appointment information should be kept in a place not easily accessible to other patients, and telephone calls that might reveal sensitive information should be answered in privacy. Office personnel should be careful never to discuss patients outside of the office.[25]

Poor patient compliance should also be noted in the record, along with any attempts by the physician to remedy the situation. Instances of missed or cancelled appointments and failure to take properly prescribed medications are examples of behavior that should be recorded. After repeated episodes of noncompliant conduct on the part of the patient, a letter should be sent (certified mail, with return receipt requested) outlining the medical consequences of such behavior, with a copy of the letter kept with the record. Consideration should be given to terminating the doctor–patient relationship with patients who consistently fail to follow proper medical advice.

Information from the medical record should be released only after a properly executed written release is received from the patient or the patient's representative. Information given over the telephone should be carefully considered, because it is impossible to know for certain who is on the other end. Certain medical information, such as drug or alcohol abuse problems or HIV status, may be protected by special rules that require specific permission for release.

LABORATORY TESTS

Laboratory results and consultation reports should be reviewed and initialed by the physician before they are placed in the medical record. It is critical that office staff not be permitted to file this material before it has been evaluated, because many instances of malpractice liability arise from mishandling this type of information. If tests are suggested in the record (i.e., "fields next visit"), they should be performed as scheduled or the reason for non-performance clearly documented.

TELEPHONE CALLS

Telephone calls from patients require special care. Often, advice given or treatment prescribed over the phone never makes it into the patient's record.

A system should be set up to be certain that all telephone calls are logged into the patient chart and that an accurate description of what took place is preserved. Even seemingly routine items such as appointment cancellations and drug refills must be carefully documented. Staff can be allowed to answer commonly asked questions as long as they are acting within the scope of their training.

PHOTOGRAPHS

Photographs of trauma, strabismus, and plastics cases are often invaluable in the defense of a medical malpractice action. These should be accurately identified and dated and should be kept with the medical record when possible. Patients shown this reminder of their preoperative condition are often less inclined to pursue legal solutions to postoperative problems.

SECOND OPINIONS

Patients often ask for second opinions and such requests should be duly noted in the chart. Never refuse a patient request for a second opinion in elective cases, and even in emergencies the request should be honored if at all possible. Second opinions create a "win–win" situation. If your opinion is corroborated the patient gains added confidence in your abilities. If you were incorrect the patient is spared possible harm, and an educational rather than a potentially confrontational situation is created. It is even useful to help the patient arrange the second opinion so that the choice of consultant will be most appropriate. When at all possible, those chosen to render second opinions should have no financial connection with your own practice.

IN THE EVENT OF A MALPRACTICE ACTION

Even a careful and competent physician may be faced at some point with malpractice litigation. Sometimes the situation will represent a legitimate claim, and at other times nothing more than a nuisance action. Each event should be taken seriously and proper steps followed, both to protect your interests and to comply with the terms of your malpractice insurance policy.

The general requirements of your malpractice policy should be understood before a potential case arises. In most instances physicians must notify the carrier if a situation occurs that could potentially lead to malpractice litigation. This may simply be a disgruntled patient or a more serious problem. Most companies do not penalize a physician who reports such a situation as long as the event does not lead to actual litigation. You should notify the carrier by certified mail—return receipt requested—and follow their instructions.

The attorney for the patient often will call and ask for an "informal conversation" just to help "straighten things out." It is usually unwise to participate in such a conversation. In no instance should a talk take place without written authorization from the patient, since breach of patient confidentiality can later be claimed. Additional specific advice and permission from your own carrier should be obtained before proceeding.

Make no promises to the patient and do not discuss liability or negligence with the patient or the patient's representative. No compensation for a complication should be suggested, even if you think you might actually have been at fault. Let the insurance company handle this type of negotiation for you.

Once an actual malpractice suit has been filed, it is important to secure the medical record. Make several copies and keep the original in a secure place. In addition, check to be certain that hospital and/or outpatient surgical records are available, and that x-rays, laboratory results, and any other relevant materials are protected. Create a diary outlining all of your thoughts and recollections concerning the case and keep it separate from the medical record so that it is not subject to subpoena as a part of that record.

Never alter the medical record. There are no exceptions to this rule. An altered record can result in loss of a defensible case because it raises damaging questions regarding the integrity of the physician. Even when an error is detected or when the record seems extremely incriminating, it is easier to try to explain what was written than to explain why it was altered. Plaintiffs' attorneys often obtain copies of hospital and other records well in advance of filing a case, and it is quite simple to detect differences between copies obtained at different times. As noted previously, errors in the record can be corrected when they are detected, but the original version should remain readable and the initials of the physician and date of the change should be clearly noted.

It is also important to cooperate with the attorney provided by the carrier. Honesty, openness, and trust in the relationship are essential. If a mistake was made it is important to acknowledge that fact. It is very important that no surprises occur. Often you must educate the attorney about the medical facts important for the case, but the attorney should be allowed to develop the legal strategy for the defense. If you feel that the attorney is not competent or if a significant personality conflict develops, discuss this with the carrier. If you have any doubt, it is usually worthwhile to hire your own attorney to represent your interests, even though this is officially the responsibility of the insurance carrier.

The settlement provisions in your policy should be carefully evaluated. Some companies may settle without your consent; others will require your permission. The decision of whether or not to settle the case may be clear-cut in some situations but quite difficult in others. Many times a physician will refuse to settle a case that really should not reach the courtroom; insurance companies also can misjudge situations and offer incorrect advice. Both parties need to put forth a good-faith effort in each case, and the cooperation of all parties is needed to come to the best resolution. If you are concerned that the advice given by your carrier may not be in your best interests, arrange for your own experienced malpractice attorney to evaluate the situation.

It is also important that the family, office staff, and other patients of the physician not bear the burden of the malpractice action. Physicians must try to maintain a relatively even keel despite the emotional stress involved. A videotape has been developed for physicians and their families to help ease the burden of this stressful situation.[26] Those involved in a malpractice situation may benefit from viewing it.

THE OPHTHALMOLOGIST AS EXPERT WITNESS

The Board of Directors of the AAO has approved a policy statement regarding presentation of expert testimony by ophthalmologists.[27] It emphasizes that it is the duty of ophthalmologists to cooperate in the judicial process by providing testimony that is "objective, truthful, and accurate," thereby assisting the jury in distinguishing between a poor medical outcome that is the result of substandard care and one that is not. It is permissible to accept reasonable payment for serving as an expert, as long as the fee is not contingent on the outcome of the case.

The witness should be familiar with the standard of care existing at the time of the event and should confine testimony regarding standards to the practices prevalent at that time. No negligence is involved in the selection of a given treatment if it was within the standard of care at the time, even if, in retrospect, an alternate choice may have been better.

4 | STARTING AND DEVELOPING A PRACTICE

Previous sections of this book make it clear that in the future ophthalmologists will face the difficult problem of increasing regulation of their practices, combined with decreasing reimbursement, fewer patients, and rising costs. This will place a premium on the optimally run practice for both the practitioner and the patient.

It will become more difficult to survive economically in a practice that fails to recognize and adjust to this new reality. At present, for the first time in recent memory, practices that have kept gross income and net profits on a steady level are regarded as having done well, since many others are actually experiencing net decreases in revenue. Those practices that are most efficient will be best able to weather the storm. Those with excessive overhead and with inefficient billing and collection systems will find themselves struggling to survive, and some will fail.

It is also likely that in the future there will be fewer and fewer solo practitioners because of the setup costs involved and the difficulty of keeping expenses low enough. This section is designed to assist you in learning how to develop and sustain a well-run practice. It will be applicable whether you are starting your own practice or joining an established physician or group. Not all suggestions are relevant to all situations; you should pick and choose the ones most appropriate for your particular circumstances.

Space constraints prevent an in-depth discussion of many important topics. There are, however, a number of excellent sources from which more extensive information can be obtained. Some of the more useful ones are listed in the annotated bibliography section on practice management at the end of this book.

EVALUATING ESTABLISHED PRACTICE OPPORTUNITIES

Whether you purchase an established practice or join as an associate, the ability to determine the actual value of the practice is extremely important. If you are becoming an associate you must determine whether or not the practice can sustain a new associate. If you are buying in, you must establish that the price you are being asked to pay is fair and reasonable. Outright purchase also demands the ability to determine a fair purchase price. Certain ground rules are applicable under both sets of circumstances and are discussed below.

PRACTICE LOAD

It is important to know how busy the practice really is. To determine this, more than the number of weeks of advance booking must be considered. The additional factors include the number of patients seen per office day, surgical load (both in absolute numbers and as a percentage of patients seen), and the source of patients seen.

Considering only the weeks of advance booking can be extremely misleading. The absolute number of patients waiting to be cared for is much more important than the weeks booked in advance because the financial impact on the practice will depend more on the former than on the latter. In addition, once the backlog is made up (regardless of the number of patients involved) there must be additional patients to fill the void or you will suddenly be very idle. All numbers should be analyzed over several years to allow a more accurate evaluation of any trend.

The percentage of patients in managed care situations also must be determined, because they will all be lost if the third-party payor removes the practice from the panel at the end of a contract year. Replacement of these patients may prove difficult under the present economic conditions.

FEES AND COLLECTIONS

The fee structure of the practice should also be analyzed, with actual charges and amount collected considered as separate items. Charges should be investigated to see if the fee structure is within the customary range for the area. A fee structure that is too low may be difficult for a new practitioner to overcome, because a sudden elevation of charges by an unknown, relatively inexperienced practitioner may cause patients to take their business elsewhere.

Payments (amount of charges actually collected) should also be analyzed. Many practices routinely write off a significant portion of their charges because of such things as various third-party payor contractual commitments and Medicare nonallowed amounts, and these amounts should be subtracted from the actual charges to determine how much income is potentially collectible. This figure, when compared with the actual amount collected, defines the collection ratio, which for most successful ophthalmic practices is over 90%.

The source of payments is also very important. A practice that derives a large percentage of its revenue from a single managed care plan is vulnerable to both the solvency of the particular insurer and its payment patterns. In addition, there is the possibility of losing the contract to another provider, which can be financially devastating. Therefore, it is unwise for a single payor, with the possible exception of Medicare, to be responsible for more than 15% of practice revenue.

Medicare, which for many ophthalmic practices is the primary source of revenue, presently reimburses new physicians at a rate significantly lower than that for established practitioners in the area. This difference, initially 20%, can decrease income substantially, especially when assignment of Medicare claims is taken. Therefore, your revenue flow may be less than that of an established practitioner even when both office and surgical volume remain constant.

In addition to the areas discussed above, the fiscal integrity of the practice should be determined. It is easy to be distracted by the size of the gross charges of a practice and even more so by the amount actually collected. However, the simple fact that large sums of money flow through a practice does not guarantee that the practice is actually profitable.

Practices have both assets and liabilities. Assets are items that contribute to the worth of the business, and liabilities are items that must be subtracted from the value. The difference, called the book value, gives a rough estimate of the overall health of the practice.

Assets include accounts receivable (money due from patients or insurance companies), the value of equipment and furnishings, leasehold improvements, and cash on hand. Liabilities include such things as accounts payable (money owed by the practice to some other entity), leases for office space and equipment, and tax and pension obligations that must be paid.

Expenses can also be categorized as fixed or variable, and the difference is important. Fixed expenses are those that cannot be easily reduced even if the practice would like to do so. These include loan and lease payments, utilities, insurance premiums, and pension plan obligations. High fixed expenses can cripple any business, especially in the face of decreasing reimbursement.

Variable expenses are those over which an individual practice has more control. These include staffing costs, benefit packages, office expenses, and similar items. In times of fiscal difficulty some of these costs can often be reduced or eliminated to reduce practice overhead. In attempting to assess the financial health of a practice, efforts should be made to consider carefully all variable costs and to determine which can be decreased by more efficient office management. This can increase the net income of the practice without the need for additional revenue.

A personal relationship with a bank is very important. Physicians use banking facilities for depositing practice funds and as a source of capital for practice development and expansion. In general, physicians are good credit risks and should be well treated by banks. Try to establish a personal relationship with an influential bank officer. You will then be dealing with someone who not only can make decisions but also has a working knowledge of your practice and its needs.

Most banks require submission of a personal financial statement as well as a viable business plan before any loans are made. Careful attention to the preparation of these documents before the money is actually required will go a long way towards ensuring prompt availability of sufficient funds when they are needed. The business plan should demonstrate that the projected cash flow of the practice will be sufficient to repay the borrowed funds. To assist new practitioners, repayment plans can be structured to allow a grace period before any payments are due and also to provide for interest-only payments for a period of time.

Rather than reapplying for a loan each time additional capital is required, it is often helpful to establish a line of credit against which loans can be taken as desired. If possible, try to avoid using personal assets (e.g., home, stocks) as collateral for business-related activities; the assets of the business in most instances should be more than adequate to provide protection for the lender.

FINANCIAL HEALTH OF THE PRACTICE

SOURCES OF FUNDS FOR PRACTICE DEVELOPMENT

Both commercial banks and thrifts (savings and loans, credit unions, mutual saving banks) are suitable sources of funds. Medical equipment distributors may also make money available, although they usually require that purchases be made from them, and care must be taken that the prices charged are competitive. Finance companies should be used only as a last resort, because they are primarily intended for high-risk borrowers and this fact is reflected in the interest rates charged.

PURCHASE OF A PRACTICE

The outright purchase of a practice, usually from a retiring physician, may be an excellent way for a new practitioner to begin. Purchase involves the acquisition of the hard assets of the practice, including equipment, supplies, leasehold improvements, charts, and records. These can usually be valued by means of a formula that takes into account the age and condition of the equipment and improvements, the depreciated value, and the replacement cost. If necessary, an equipment broker or practice management consultant can be enlisted to provide a fair value for these assets.

The information needed to evaluate properly a potential purchase can usually be obtained from several readily available sources. If the practice is a sole proprietorship, the information on business income and expenses can be obtained from Schedule C of the individual federal income tax return. Partnerships and corporations file separate returns that contain the same information. Several years' worth of returns should be reviewed so that any trends can be adequately evaluated. If you are unwilling or feel unable to perform such a review, find an advisor with the requisite knowledge and experience. Not all accountants and attorneys possess the expertise to perform this service.

Accounts receivable, another asset of the practice, may or may not be included in the purchase price, because their true value is often difficult to assess. Frequently they are retained by the seller and a fee is paid to the purchaser of the practice to assist with collection. If the decision is made for the purchaser to acquire the accounts receivable also, their value should be reduced to the amount actually collectible by considering such factors as their age and discounts for Medicare and other third-party payors.

GOODWILL

An important additional consideration is the goodwill value of the practice. The concept of goodwill, and especially how much to pay for it when a practice or a share of a practice is purchased, is one of the most troublesome and misunderstood aspects of practice acquisition. Goodwill has been defined as the ongoing value of an established practice resulting from previous efforts of the owners. It includes the location of the practice, its reputation in the community, patient population, and business efficiency. In essence, it is the amount in excess of the value of the "hard assets" that is added to the purchase price to compensate the owner for past efforts expended in developing a better product.

Various formulas have been suggested as guidelines for goodwill evaluation (e.g., 44% of last year's gross, excess earnings value over the average ophthalmic practice), but all of them, although useful in providing rough guidelines, are inadequate for comparing individual practices that may widely vary in quality and growth potential despite certain superficial similarities. Thus, two practices with the same gross earnings may actually have very different goodwill values because of other important considerations.

The following example may make this more clear. Consider the two hypothetical practices described in Fig. 4.1. According to many of the usual formulas, the goodwill values of the two practices would be similar. Even a cursory analysis of the information provided, however, indicates that such a conclusion is probably not reasonable. Indeed, it is often more useful to look at the goodwill payment as an opportunity cost for the privilege of securing a particular practice as opposed to a different one, or even starting from scratch. In other words, how much of a premium am I willing to pay to acquire this particular business compared with all others?

If goodwill is calculated in this fashion, rather than by a strict formula, each practice can be assessed in the same way as any other business investment. An investment opportunity that is expected to yield better than average returns in the future usually demands a higher premium initially.

To assist in this process, the "book value" of each practice should be determined. This allows comparison of the true "nuts and bolts" value of each opportunity. The approximate cost of starting a practice from scratch in the same area should next be estimated. Factors that make a particular practice better or worse than average should then be considered. These include location, growth rate, reputation in the community, fee structure, and managed care contract status. By using this or a similar method, each practice opportunity can be ranked objectively and compared with the other available options. The goodwill payment asked in each situation can then be compared with the practice rating to see if the sum proposed is reasonable. When this is done, an amount that initially seems unreasonable may prove not to be so; conversely, some seemingly moderate fees will be demonstrated to be outrageous.

If you decide to join an ongoing practice rather than to brave it alone, some type of written contract is needed to define carefully the duties and responsibilities of all parties. It is important to insist on a written contract and not simply a "handshake agreement," so that both the employer and employee are properly protected. The contract should represent an accurate and com-

JOINING A PRACTICE
CONTRACT CONSIDERATIONS

Figure 4.1. Hypothetical Practices for Evaluation of Goodwill

	PRACTICE A	PRACTICE B
1992 Gross income	$500,000	$500,000
1991 Gross income	$400,000	$500,000
1990 Gross income	$300,000	$480,000
1992 Surgery load	125 Cataracts	125 Cataracts
1991 Surgery load	95	120
1990 Surgery load	75	120
Patient total 1992/1991	+20%	+2%
Book value	$250,000	$250,000
Goodwill value	?	?

plete description of all oral agreements. Therefore, all parties should understand that the written provisions of the contract replace any and all previous orally defined stipulations. The contract should be reviewed by an attorney—not just a practice management advisor—familiar with the laws of the state in which the contract will be enforced, and should be clearly understood by all parties before it is signed. The advisors for the prospective employee should be different from those used by the employer, to avoid possible conflicts of interest. Attorneys, accountants, and practice management advisors with experience in reviewing medical contracts (especially those of ophthalmic practices) should be sought, because their advice is likely to be the most valuable.

The form of the contract can vary widely; it may be a simple letter of understanding or a more complex document many pages long. Either model is sufficient as long as all important points are covered. Items defined in any contract should include duties, salary considerations, benefits, restrictive covenant if applicable, future buy-in formula, and termination procedures. In fact, from the point of view of the new employee, the most important consideration may be adequate protection in the event employment is terminated. Proper notice, severance pay, continuation of insurance and other benefits, access to patient records, return of monies paid for buy-in, and malpractice tail premium payment are issues that should be addressed. Evaluate the value of the package as a whole and do not be misled by overly attractive initial salary offers. In some instances, the higher the initial salary, the less attractive the offer is over the long term.

Most physicians have little experience in negotiating contracts, and the process can be trying for both employer and employee. Willingness to compromise, especially on nonessential issues, is important if the process is to be successfully concluded. Contracts that are grossly unfair to either party are unlikely to result in the stable relationship that should be the goal of all negotiations. Both sides should rank their objectives in order of importance and should be willing to compromise on items near the bottom of their respective lists.

RESTRICTIVE COVENANTS

More and more, restrictive covenants are becoming a part of employment contracts. This is done by employers to protect their patient base in the event the employee leaves. Although some states prohibit such restrictions, most do not, and these "covenants not to compete" are usually enforceable if they are reasonable in scope. In particular, if enforcement of the covenant does not pose a threat to the general health of the community, it is likely to be upheld.

Even covenants that contain an absolute prohibition against competition usually cannot prevent the physician from opening a practice in a given location if he or she wishes to do so. The real purpose of a covenant is to compensate the injured party (i.e., the former employer) for economic damages caused by such action taken in violation of a contractual agreement. Because the argument in most instances is primarily about money, protracted and expensive litigation can often be avoided by specifying a "liquidating amount" payable by the employee to the employer in the event that provisions of the covenant are violated.

If this mechanism is chosen, the business necessity for the covenant should be clearly stated in the contract and the basis for the calculation of the amount of liquidating damages carefully defined. This amount should be determined by estimating the actual economic damage the former employer will suffer; it is important that the amount reflect a careful assessment and not represent an arbitrarily chosen, strictly punitive amount. If the latter occurs, the agreement is more likely to be rejected by the courts.[1]

Contracts may also contain "nonsolicitation" provisions in addition to noncompete stipulations. These restrict the employee from approaching the patients of the practice and also existing hospital, HMO, PPO, nursing home, and other contract sources. They are often dealt with in a similar fashion to the noncompete clause. The law in this area is confusing and is constantly changing. Therefore, accurate up-to-date information about this problem should be obtained at the time any contract is being considered.

RUNNING A SUCCESSFUL PRACTICE
FINANCE

The key to running a successful practice is to assemble a team of talented and experienced advisors. These professionals can provide invaluable advice on legal and fiscal matters and are important members of the management team. Not all practices will require each of these individuals, for often one person can provide assistance in several areas. Because their services are not inexpensive, a thorough understanding of the fee structure for all consultants is mandatory, with costs agreed on before they are hired. Most of these professionals, unlike physicians, bill on the basis of time spent (including telephone time), so idle chitchat should be kept to a minimum. Know the questions you want answered before you make the call.

An experienced attorney is essential to a well-run practice. The attorney should review all leases, contracts, and other important documents before they are signed. Information on tax and retirement plans should also be available. Recent changes in federal and state law concerning employment practices, age and sex discrimination, sexual harassment in the workplace, and exposure to occupational hazards make access to advice in these areas essential as well. Those in a group practice should obtain advice from an independent attorney for matters concerning specific interactions with the group.

An accountant familiar with medical practice and small business management is also very important. This individual, who should be a certified public accountant (CPA), will provide a method for evaluating the financial health of the practice, controls to ensure accurate record keeping, and audit trails to prevent embezzlement. Preparation of the various tax returns required of the practice should be included. References for all candidates should be obtained and checked carefully. Experience with medical office accounting should be a primary consideration.

Often the accountant can teach selected employees some of the simpler bookkeeping functions, helping to reduce accounting costs. A bookkeeper can also be hired to provide some services at lower cost than the accountant.

Hiring an accountant does not relieve the physician of the ultimate responsibility for overseeing the financial aspects of the practice; it merely provides assistance. In fact, an interested physician who regularly reviews collections, billings, day sheets, and the checking account is a much better deterrent to theft from the practice than the most diligent accountant.

Ophthalmologists hire more management consultants than any other specialty. These consultants can provide assistance with office management, practice marketing, scheduling, and various other tasks outside the expertise of most lawyers and accountants. Many excellent publications are also available to assist in this very important area. Because of the special needs of most ophthalmic practices, consultants with experience in ophthalmology should be actively sought.*

BASIC OFFICE MANAGEMENT

Running a medical office is not really different from running a small business. Medical practices are really service businesses, with success dependent on continually pleasing the patients and providing the products and services that they desire. Systems must be in place to ensure that patients have the opportunity to be seen by the practice, to be treated appropriately, to be charged a reasonable fee for the services provided, and to be scheduled for future appointments as needed. Ancillary products, such as glasses or contact lenses, can be ethically dispensed on site for both the convenience of the patient and the financial benefit of the practice.

The concepts of total quality management (TQM) and continuous quality improvement (CQI), although primarily applicable to manufacturing processes, can help to improve medical office practices as well.[2] Perhaps the most important lesson is to focus on improving the process of office managment rather than berating individuals when problems develop. There is an understandable tendency to blame the person when quality control breaks down, but experience indicates that most of the time the process is really to blame. Involving everyone in the attempt to improve the process—with the team philosophy of "*How* can we fix it?" rather than "*Who* can we blame?"—encourages cooperation rather than confrontation.

Treating patients, vendors, nurses, and hospital personnel as partners rather than "customers" is often of tremendous value. These are all excellent potential sources of referrals, and will usually tend to recommend those who treat them with respect and understanding. In a service business, the perception of quality is often just as important as the reality, a point that should always be kept in mind.

An example might be a patient who damages a new soft contact lens within a week of getting it after not needing one previously for 2 years. The patient is convinced that the contact "must have been defective," although the more likely explanation is that the patient was really at fault. Arguments will just make the patient feel more victimized; giving the patient another contact lens without argument solves the problem at very little cost and enhances the reputation of the practice in the eyes of the patient. In turn, a sympathetic product representative can be approached about getting a free replacement or allowance, reducing the actual cost to the practice even further.

Perhaps the key lesson from the CQI–TQM philosophy is the concept of improving processes from the "front end" rather than after problems have occurred. This involves analysis of all office procedures and policies, even those that seem to be working well, to see if there is some way they can be made even better. Although "if it ain't broke, don't fix it" is often the most reasonable course of action, CQI–TQM encourages you at least to take a peek!

---

*The American Academy of Ophthalmology has a list of experienced consultants available, and additional information can also be obtained from the Society of Professional Business Consultants (621 Plainfield, Suite 308, Willowbrook, IL, 60521).

A policy and personnel manual is an important part of an office practice. As noted by employment attorney Peter Harris Rudy,[3] it should represent an up-to-date compilation of the rules and regulations under which the office runs. It covers such areas as definitions of benefits (e.g., vacation, sick leave, personal leave), rules of conduct, policies on discrimination and sexual harassment, and other matters. "Employer writings" such as handbooks have been increasingly involved in litigation concerning the contractual obligations of employers to employees. Nevertheless, it is probably safer to have than not to have one because, in the absence of a written policy, oral representations of policy and procedures can be contractually binding and very difficult to refute. Once litigation ensues there is a presumption that the handbook will be one of the elements on which the decisions will be made.

The major advantage of a handbook is that all of the materials can be reviewed before they are made available to employees. Employment policies (and employment law) are evolving areas, and attention to changes and regular review of the document by the practice attorney are essential.

Some of the key factors to be considered in constructing a manual for your office are:

1. Do we really mean it?
2. Do we really do this?
3. Do we need to state this in writing?
4. Will employees (supervisors) understand this?
5. Is there a better way to do or say this?
6. Do we need to put in limiting language?
7. Do we need to preserve management discretion in this area?

In addition to the professional advisors and consultants discussed earlier, it is necessary to staff the office with competent employees. These are the people that the patients deal with on a day-to-day basis, and their ability and personality can make or break a practice. This makes the selection process especially important.

It is sometimes difficult to decide exactly how many employees are really needed. Overhead costs are ever increasing, and too many employees for the work available constitutes one possible source of unnecessary expense. On the other hand, enough people must be available to ensure that all of the needs of the patients and practice can be satisfied.

To assist in making hiring decisions, it is helpful to draft an office staffing plan with job descriptions for all the important tasks that must be performed. A job description defines the purpose of the job, the knowledge and skills necessary, licensure requirements, supervision available, and any special physical or experience criteria to be satisfied. It makes clear to all exactly what is expected, and can also include salary and benefits provided. With proper planning and guidance, one employee can often accomplish many individual jobs and still function efficiently.

It is important that any tests required to secure a given position be relevant to those tasks necessary to perform the job in a satisfactory manner. Tests not relevant to job performance and that may exclude otherwise qualified individuals—especially women, minorities, and the handicapped—are both illegal and unfair, and may subject the practice to legal challenge.

POLICY AND PERSONNEL MANUAL

OFFICE PERSONNEL

HIRING CONSIDERATIONS

Prospective employees can be found by word of mouth, classified ads placed by the practice, or from employment agencies. The latter method is the most expensive and should be avoided if possible. Hiring workers currently employed by hospitals and other practitioners in the area is another option, but you will not be very popular if this method is used frequently. Part-time employees are often quite useful for specific tasks, and usually are accorded far fewer fringe benefits than full-time employees, thus reducing overhead costs.[4] Job sharing can also be used to attract and/or retain skilled staff members with special family needs.

Figure 4.2. Sample Employment Application (Front)

APPLICATION FOR EMPLOYMENT

Date _______________

Name ___________________________ Soc. Sec. # ___________________
     Last   First   Middle

Present Address ____
     No.   Street   Apt.   City/State/Zip

Permanent Address ____
     No.   Street   Apt.   City/State/Zip

Phone ______________ Phone _____________ Message Phone ___________________

Position Applied For ____

Salary Desired _________________ Referred By _______________________

If your application is considered favorably, what date are you available to begin work? ____

Circle days available: M T W Th F S Su

Hours available: Days __________ Evenings __________

RECORD OF EDUCATION

	Name & Location			
Education	(City/State) of School	Years Attended	Graduate?	Major
High School				
College				
College				
Other				

Subjects of special study or research work ___________________________

____

Are you legally elegible for employment in the USA? _________________

(Proof of identity and citizenship or immigration status will be required upon employment.)

What foreign language do you speak fluently? _________________________

Read? _____________________________ Write? _______________________

Employees with experience in a particular area can be especially useful to new practitioners, who usually have little of their own on which to build. There is a risk, however, in hiring workers whose experience and training may encourage them to perform in ways that are not compatible with your own practice image. They may also be quite set in their ways and find it difficult to adjust to new ways of doing things. For example, an insurance clerk experienced with submitting paper claims may be reluctant to lead the conversion to electronic billing, even though it may be in the best interests of the practice to switch.

Only certain questions can be asked on prospective employment appli-

---

Figure 4.2. Sample Employment Application (Back)

PREVIOUS EMPLOYMENT
(LAST THREE POSITIONS HELD)

Mo/Year   Name & Address of Employer   Position Title & Job Description

From: ____

To: ____

Reason for Leaving ____

From: ____

To: ____

Reason for Leaving ____

From: ____

To: ____

Reason for Leaving ____

Are there other experiences or skills which would particularly qualify you for work with our organization? ____

Have you ever been bonded? _________ If yes, on what jobs? _____________

Are you willing to work overtime if required? _________________________

Have you ever been convicted of a felony? ___________________________

If yes, describe in full ____

Do you have any physical condition which may limit your ability to perform the job applied for? ____

If yes, describe in full ____

This document does not constitute an employment contract. Employment is at the will of both the employer and each employee and may be terminated by either.

I certify that all information provided above is true and complete and that any misrepresentation may subject me to disqualification or dismissal. I authorize the verification of the above by this office as required and authorize my previous employers to release to the company the information requested.

Signature ____ Date ____________

(Reproduced by permission from *The Guide.*)

cations. A satisfactory form is shown in Figure 4.2. All applicants should be asked to complete the form before the employment interview and to sign a release allowing the prospective employer to contact previous employers, references, and others necessary to verify the information listed on the application. Anyone who refuses to sign such a release should probably not be hired.

JOB INTERVIEW

Only applicants whose preliminary resumé seems promising should have a personal interview. As with the employment application, there are certain questions that are not permissible before an employee is hired. Some of these are outlined in Fig. 4.3. Additional prohibitions related to the Americans with Disabilities Act (discussed below) have recently been instituted. However, it is possible to gather a lot of useful information about prospective employees even with these limitations. Important questions to ask include why they would like the position, what special skills they would bring to the

Figure 4.3. Permissible and Nonpermissible Employment Interview Questions

SUBJECT	ACCEPTABLE QUESTIONS	UNNACCEPTABLE QUESTIONS
Name	For access purposes, whether applicant's work records are under another name.	To ask if female applicant is Miss, Mrs., or Ms., or to ask for maiden name.
Residence	Place and length of current and previous addresses. Applicant's phone number or how applicant can be reached.	Whether applicant owns or rents.
Age	Before hiring (if doubtful from applicant's appearance) whether age 16 or older. After hiring, proof of age by birth certificate.	Age or age group of applicant. Birth certificate or baptismal record for hiring.
National origin	None, except for business necessity.	Birthplace of applicant, parents, grandparents, or spouse. Any other inquiry into national origin.
Race	Statistics on race for affirmative action plan *after hiring*.	Any inquiry that would indicate race or color.
Sex	Inquiry for affirmative action plan statistics *after hiring*.	Inquiry that would indicate sex unless job related.
Religion	None, except for employer that is a religious institution.	Religion or religious customs and holidays. Recommendations or references from church officials.
Citizenship	Federal Form I-9 required.	Any questions not on Federal Form I-9.
Marital status	Status (only married or single) <I>after hiring<I> for insurance and tax purposes. Number and ages of children <I>after hiring<I> for insurance and tax purposes.	To ask marital status before hiring. To ask the number and ages of children and who cares for them, or if applicant plans to have children.

job, and why they think they should be hired. You should also try to determine why they are looking for a new opportunity, and what they liked most and least about their former (or current) job. After the interview is completed, impressions regarding poise, appearance, language skills, maturity, and other factors should be noted as well.

Unless the situation is unusual, the applicant should not be hired on the spot so that others can be evaluated and references properly checked. Once all applicants have been interviewed, they should be formally ranked and the one most qualified offered the job. Those candidates not hired should be so notified in a polite letter thanking them for their interest. It is important to keep a written record of the rankings of each applicant to protect yourself from future charges of discrimination.

The person hired should be sent a formal letter outlining the job title,

Figure 4.3. Permissible and Nonpermissible Employment Interview Questions

SUBJECT	ACCEPTABLE QUESTIONS	UNNACCEPTABLE QUESTIONS
Physical data	To require applicant to prove ability to do manual labor, lifting, and other physical requirements of the job, if any. Require a physical examination.	To ask height and weight, impairment, or other nonspecified job-related physical data.
Handicap	To inquire for the purpose of determining applicant's capability to perform the job. (Burden of proof for nondiscrimination lies with the employer.)	To exclude or not reasonably accommodate handicapped applicants as a class on the basis of their type of handicap. Each case must be determined individually.
Other qualifications	Any area that has a direct reflection on the job applied for.	Any non-job-related inquiry that may present information permitting unlawful discrimination.

THE INTERVIEW

The type of questions you may ask during a job interview is limited but this does not preclude an in-depth interview to obtain information you need. Below are sample questions to help you conduct the interview. Answers to these questions will help determine the applicant's ability to fill your job position.

1. What is your primary reason for wanting this position?
2. Why are you looking for a new position?
3. Which of your previous jobs did you like the best? Why?
4. What did you like most/least about your last position?
5. What was a typical day like in your previous position?
6. Where do you see yourself in the next five years?
7. What is your greatest strength? Weakness?
8. How do you feel about working overtime on occasion?
9. Do you have any questions about the job description or what we have talked about?

Reproduced by permission from *The Guide*.

salary, and date to report. The letter should emphasize that the employment is not for a specific term and that it can be terminated at any time by either party with or without cause—so-called "at will" employment. A copy of the office policy and procedures manual should be given to the newcomer and used as a reference for further information about the office.

WAGES AND BENEFITS

Fair wage and benefit packages are necessary to attract and keep high-quality employees. Appropriate salary levels for office personnel vary tremendously from area to area and should be at the high end of the scale if you expect to keep talented personnel. It is much wiser and far less disruptive to pay valued employees slightly more than you need to rather than to risk their departure for a better offer. Patients like familiar faces, and the stability that long-term employees give an office is invaluable.

SALARY

Salary is the basic cash compensation that employees receive. It can be computed on an hourly, weekly, or monthly basis, with federal, state, and local income taxes and social security taxes usually withheld by the employer. The salary policy and range for the job should be defined in advance, and increases should be based primarily on performance rather than longevity. Bonuses given at certain times of the year such as Christmas quickly become expected by employees and are difficult to discontinue once started. For that reason, alternate forms of incentive compensation should be used whenever possible.

Almost all employees in medical offices are eligible for both overtime compensation and minimum wage levels, regardless of how their basic salary is computed. Only executives and administrators who spend more than 60% of their time directing others in their work, and professional staff such as MDs, RNs, and PAs, are customarily exempt. Overtime takes effect when more than 40 hours of work are performed in a given week, and federal law requires compensation at a rate 1.5 base salary level. For that reason, office policy should require approval from a supervisor before overtime is permitted. Compensatory time off in lieu of salary can be given during the same pay period if the employee agrees, but must be given at the same salary rate as cash overtime compensation.

Physicians often place significant demands on employees in terms of hours worked and assume that those employees are just as happy to work late as they are. That is often not the case, and repeatedly ignoring the family and personal responsibilities of employees may result in the loss of a valuable team member.

The burden of proof regarding hours worked rests with the employer, and a mechanism, such as a time clock or a sign-in sheet, should be in place in all offices to document accurately this number for each employee. Lunch hour policies should be clearly defined, because eating while working is defined as work for purposes of overtime compensation. State law may be even more favorable to employees than federal law, and good legal advice is essential to avoid potential problems.

BENEFITS

Granted in addition to salary, the so-called "fringe benefits" have become more important in recent years. They offer advantages to employees in that their value is frequently not taxable as income, and the employer benefits as well because they are still considered a tax-deductible business expense. Some of the more common benefits are listed in Figure 4.4. It is sometimes possible to offer a "cafeteria package" of benefits by giving each employee a given dollar amount to spend and having the employee design the package that is most useful in his particular case. Some employees, for example, might wish assistance with day care expenses rather than health care coverage that might be redundant if their spouses are employed.

Detailed descriptions of the various fringe benefits should be available in your office policy and procedures manual. This book should be revised when changes are made so that it remains accurate and up to date. Because this volume can be used by both employees and employers to resolve disputes, do not include anything in it that will not be beneficial to the practice.

PERFORMANCE REVIEWS

All employees should have a formal assessment of their performance by their supervisor at least once a year. This is necessary to provide the employee with information needed to correct problems that have occurred as well as to acknowledge areas of exceptional achievement. The review should be done in standardized fashion and should be as free from personal bias as possible. Sometimes it is also helpful to ask the employee to evaluate his or her own performance and to see how it differs from the supervisor's evaluation. Employees should sign the evaluation (which indicates only that it was reviewed) and be permitted to make comments for inclusion in their permanent personnel file. Office policy should allow employees with grievances to be heard by a different supervisor or by the physician personally.

Substandard performance that fails to improve should be carefully documented and penalties discussed with the employee. Repeated failures to correct deficiencies should be noted, along with warnings given regarding the time and effort needed to correct the problem and the deadline for doing so. If improvement is not forthcoming, the penalties that were defined should be imposed—otherwise, it may be difficult to dismiss the employee without

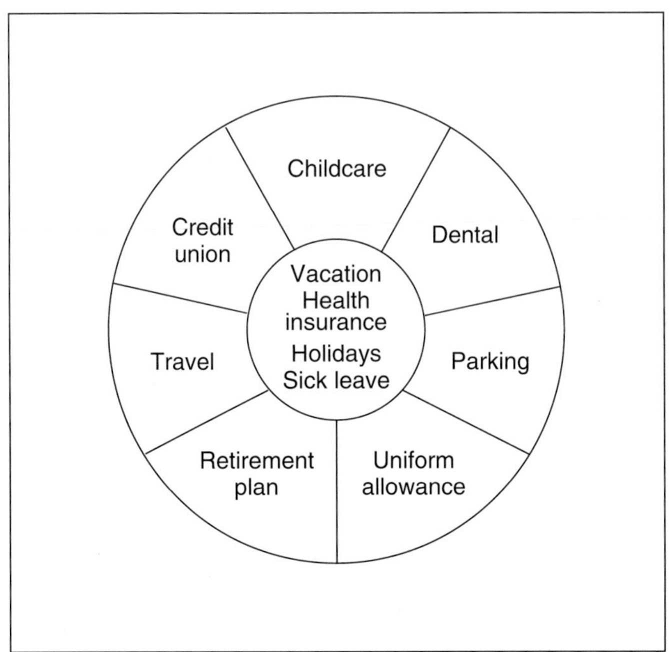

4.4 | Frequently offered fringe benefits. Core benefits are in the inner circle; flexible benefits, in the outer circle.

running the risk of legal challenge. Copies of all of the aforementioned transactions should be maintained in the personnel file.

TERMINATION

Unfortunately, it may become necessary to terminate an employee whose performance remains unsatisfactory despite all efforts to improve it. Firing an employee is never easy, but the continued presence of an unacceptable staff member can disrupt an entire office. When an employee is dismissed for cause, the final paycheck should be ready and should include all vacation, sick leave, and other accrued benefits, as well as the salary due. All keys, passes, identification cards, and other appropriate materials should be obtained from the employees before they leave. On-the-spot dismissals are usually unwise, unless the transgression is so grave that the further presence of the individual can no longer be tolerated.

Termination of employees must be handled carefully to avoid later charges of discrimination. The actual process should be as straightforward as possible. From the beginning, it should be indicated that the decision is final, the reason(s) should be clearly documented and calmly presented, and no debate or argument should be permitted. Be certain that the reason for dismissal does not relate to the race, sex, age, national origin, religion, marital status, or physical handicap of the employee. Involve your practice attorney from the beginning if the situation has the potential to become complicated. The former employee may be eligible for unemployment compensation even if his or her performance was unsatisfactory in your eyes.

If employees wish to resign voluntarily, their written resignations should be accepted and kept in the personnel file. If the employees are willing, exit interviews may be useful to help avoid the same mistake from occurring again. In addition, exit interviews with employees that leave under more pleasant circumstances (e.g., moving, promotions) may result in improved training methods and job descriptions, and may enhance the performance of the next employee.

INDEPENDENT CONTRACTORS

There is a tremendous temptation to classify workers as independent contractors rather than employees. For employees, the employer must pay social security and Medicare payroll taxes, withhold and forward federal, state, and local income taxes, and frequently provide fringe benefits; the same individual, as an independent contractor, would not require the practice to incur these expenses. Since fringe benefits alone can amount to a 25% addition to the actual salary paid, the opportunity to avoid these expenses is enticing. Many individuals would also prefer to be classed as independent contractors, since they may receive greater cash compensation and be eligible for certain additional tax deductions.[5]

Unfortunately, the Internal Revenue Service has taken a hard line in defining the eligibility criteria for independent contractors, with the result that very few workers actually qualify. The IRS provides a list of 20 factors on which they base the decision. Key factors extablishing the individual as an employee include the ability of the employer to determine when, where, and how the individual does the work and payment of an hourly, weekly, or monthly wage rather than piecework. Additional elements relate to exclusive provision of services, training responsibilities, and payment of business-related expenses.[6] The net result has been to void almost all independent contractor arrangements, with the exception of individuals (such as accountants and lawyers) who maintain their own offices, equipment, insurance coverage, and telephone numbers. In addition, if an employer does not carry Workers' Compensation Insurance on an individual who is thought to be an independent contractor, and that individual is injured and later shown to be an employee, the business will be forced to pay all related costs on an out-of-pocket basis. Therefore, expert legal advice should be obtained before you decide to take the independent contractor route.[7]

All physicians, including ophthalmologists, are bound by the Occupational Safety and Health Administration (OSHA) rules for safe office handling and disposal of blood-borne pathogens and other infectious waste. The regulations, published in the Federal Register,[8] specify the definitions of the materials covered, the procedures to be followed, and the penalties for noncompliance, with fines of up to $7000 for a single violation. Unlike many federal publications, the actual text found in the Federal Register is relatively short and easy to understand, stating clearly the responsibilities of both employers and employees under the rules.

The standards, which became effective in March 1992, require that medical practices take care to protect all employees who might be exposed, in the course of performing their normal duties, to materials that could transmit hepatitis B virus or the HIV virus. In the typical ophthalmologist's office, the most likely sources of covered risk would be exposure to blood itself, skin or other biopsy specimens before they are fixed, and needles, instruments, dressings, and supplies used in minor office surgical procedures. Certain specialized practices may have additional areas of concern. Fortunately non-bloody tears are not subject to bloodborne pathogen precautions.

The key element in complying with the OSHA requirements is the presence of an Exposure Control Plan. This plan must list all of the *job classifications* in which ALL employees so classed have the potential for occupational exposure to infectious materials. A list of job classifications in which SOME employees might have exposure must also be developed. In addition, a listing of *tasks or procedures* during which exposure might occur is needed, so that employees can be properly protected while performing them.

The plan must further specify particular measures that the employee and the facility should take to minimize risks of exposure, as well as the measures to be taken if exposure does occur. It must document the training received and describe any protective equipment required. All employees at

FEDERAL REGULATIONS APPLICABLE TO OFFICE PRACTICE
BLOOD-BORNE PATHOGEN SAFETY

Figure 4.5. OSHA Blood-borne Pathogen Risk Management Categories

1. Engineering controls
2. Work practice controls
3. Personal protective equipment
4. Housekeeping chores
5. Hepatitis B vaccinations

Adapted from Anna Adler, RN, BSN, *Bloodborne Pathogen Rules,* Vail Management Institute, 1992.

risk should be instructed in the principle of observance of *universal precautions,* which presumes that all human blood and other potentially contaminated body fluids and materials must be treated as if they are known to be contaminated by infectious agents.[9]

Risk reduction is basically divided into five broad categories (Fig. 4.5).[10] *Engineering controls* include physical systems, such as self-sheathing needles, sterilizing systems, sharps disposal containers, and infectious waste disposal areas that are easily accessible and properly identified as containing biohazardous materials. *Work practice controls* include such policies as not recapping or removing needles and other potentially hazardous sharps by hand and strict handwashing after handling potentially contaminated materials, even when gloves have been worn. If handwashing facilities are not immediately available, antiseptic hand cleaning materials must be provided. Eating, drinking, and handling of contact lenses should also be avoided in areas where exposure to potentially contaminated materials may occur, and food and drinks should also not be stored where exposure to blood or other potentially infections materials may take place.

Personal protective equipment must be provided to all employees who need it at no cost, and they must be properly instructed in its use. This typically includes such things as gloves, masks, gowns, face shields, and protective eyewear, which are designed to prevent infectious materials from reaching skin or mucous membranes. It should be emphasized to employees that these devices are required to be used each time a covered task is performed, since the employer is liable if they are not and an accidental exposure occurs. Proper disposal facilities for equipment that is discarded after use must be provided. Disposable gloves are the commonest barrier equipment provided and should not be reused.

Housekeeping chores that are required include proper disposal facilities for contaminated materials and properly marked laundry bags for reusable protective equipment. Biohazard labels must be used to properly mark all infectious materials.

Hepatitis B vaccinations must also be offered at no cost to all employees at risk who are not already immune. This vaccine is more than 85% effective in preventing the development of the disease or carrier status. The current vaccines are made from yeast derivatives and have a very low rate of adverse reaction. Three injections over a 6-month period are required. Employees may decline to be vaccinated but must sign a release indicating that the risks of doing so were explained to them.

Training of employees must take place at the time of initial assignment to duties and annually thereafter. Training records must be retained for 3 years and must include dates and a summary of the information covered. Medical records of employees at risk for occupational exposure must be kept for the duration of the employment *plus 30 years.*[11]

Because of the complexity of the regulations and the process required to remain in compliance, a cottage industry has arisen to assist physicians with the task. OSHA itself makes materials available, and the AMA and AAO also have programs to assist. In addition, commercial vendors and many hospitals provide the instruction courses required for annual training. Because the penalties for noncompliance are severe, it is important that each office carefully observe the regulations and obtain advice and consultation where required. It is estimated that it will cost the average office at least $1200 on an annual basis to remain in compliance.

The Americans with Disabilities Act (ADA), which went into effect in July 1992, gives protection to individuals with disabilities similar to that already provided on the basis of age, sex, color, national origin, and religion. The meaning of *disability* under the act is both broad and ill-defined; it includes anyone who has a "physical or mental impairment that substantially limits one or more major life activities, has a record of such an impairment, or is regarded as having such an impairment." "Major life activities" are considered to include caring for oneself, performing manual tasks, seeing, speaking, breathing, and working.[12] The ADA protects those with AIDS or who are HIV positive, as well as individuals with alcoholism and drug addiction, but homosexuals and bisexuals are not included. It is estimated that 43 million Americans will be covered under the provisions.

The ADA has two provisions that apply to those in the office practice of ophthalmology. The first (Title I) deals with employment issues and, by July of 1994, will cover all practices with 15 or more employees. This provision requires employers to hire an individual with a disability if the person is the most qualified for the job and if the disability would not interfere significantly with the individual's ability to perform the essential functions of the task. It also prohibits the discharge of a current employee because of a disability if that individual can perform the essential functions of the job with or without "reasonable accommodation" being made by the employer.[13] Thus, a person confined to a wheelchair could not be discharged as a telephone receptionist but could be denied employment as a file clerk if accessability to high shelves were required and could not be easily modified. The law does not set quotas for hiring disabled individuals and does not give them preference in employment opportunities. The Equal Employment Opportunity Commission will enforce this provision under the rules applicable to Title VII of the Civil Rights Act of 1964.[12]

The ADA has also influenced other aspects of the employment relationship. Certain questions about health, disabilities, and past Workers' Compensation claims are off limits. Careful job descriptions outlining the physical requirements of each task (separating the "esential" and "marginal" elements of each assignment) are even more important than in the past to help justify decisions regarding hiring (or not hiring) disabled individuals. In addition, under the terms of the ADA, personnel records must now be kept for 12 months. These records now include application forms, applicant resumés, interview notes, and similar items, regardless of whether the applicant was actually hired.[3]

Title III concerns public accommodations for patients and applies to all offices regardless of size. Places of public accommodation must be designed, constructed, and altered to comply with the standards outlined in the law. Physicians cannot refuse to treat or accept patients because they have a disability. They can, however, decline to treat disabled individuals if the disability is not the reason for the action (e.g., not taking new patients, wrong specialty). Physical access problems must be accomodated and, in addition, "auxilliary aids" and assistance must be provided during the examination process to ensure that effective communication with patients can be established and maintained. Braille materials and qualified interpreters for the hearing impaired are two important aids that must be considered. Private parties may bring lawsuits under the ADA to demand enforcement of the provisions of the law, but no additional damages were initially available. However, in the Civil Rights Act, the ADA was actually amended to allow for imposition of additional penalties. The Attorney General may also file suit

AMERICANS WITH
DISABILITIES ACT

under certain circumstances, and in this instance both monetary damages and civil penalties can be assessed.

The details of compliance with both portions of the ADA are complicated and are well outlined in a publication provided by the AMA.[14] Additional information can also be obtained from the Department of Justice ADA Hotline (202-514-0301) and the Job Accommodation Network (800-526-7234). Competent legal advice should be obtained for assistance with specific problems.

According to a recent article[15] in the last 6 months of 1992 the EEOC received over 3,000 charges of discrimination against those with disabilities, and 2,000 more were filed by February of 1993. Almost half of these charges concerned wrongful discharge protests, with back problems being the most common alleged impairment. Less than 4% related to visual, hearing, or HIV+ issues. In addition, because most of the decisions under this act are going to be made on a case-by-case basis (due to the very individual nature of specific jobs in different offices), it will be years before a significant set of precedents is developed to allow employers to make reliable hiring decisions.[16]

THE FAMILY AND MEDICAL LEAVE ACT OF 1993 (FLMA)

This act,[17] signed into law by President Clinton with an effective date of August 1993, provides up to 12 weeks of unpaid leave per year for employees to use associated with the birth or adoption of a child or for a serious medical condition striking the employee, a parent, spouse, or child. The job of the individual is protected during this period, and health insurance benefits must be maintained and paid for by the employer as long as the employee returns to work at the end of the leave period. FLMA applies to all employers with 50 or more full-, part-time, or temporary employees and covers employees who have worked for the employer for 12 months and have worked 20 weeks in the 12 months immediately preceding the leave request. The employer may substitute paid leave for all or part of the 12-week period. Thirty-day advance notice is required when practicable.

Civil penalties are provided in the act as a penalty for employers who fail to comply, with double damages if the noncompliance is deemed to have been willful. Since the act applies primarily to "large" small businesses, its effect on the average ophthalmology practice will probably not be extensive. However, it will certainly make some employers think twice before expanding to over 50 employees, and in the future could be modified to apply to smaller practices as well.

MEDICARE FRAUD AND ABUSE: THE SAFE HARBOR RULES

After years of preparation, the final regulations for the Medicare and Medicaid Program Protection Act of 1987 were finally released in 1991.[18] These regulations provide criminal penalties for "individuals or entities that knowingly and willfully offer, pay, solicit or receive remuneration in order to induce business reimbursed under the Medicare or state health care programs." Any violation is considered a felony, with penalties of imprisonment for up to 5 years and fines as high as $25,000.

The rules proposed are vague in many instances, and often it is not clear whether or not a particular circumstance constitutes a violation. In an effort to clarify the situation, 11 so-called "safe harbors" were created. The safe harbors describe specific situations deemed to be in compliance with the rules. Presumably, the physicians who follow these provisions will be safe from enforcement actions under the act.

The safe harbors cover many areas (Fig. 4.6), including space and equipment rental, sale of practices, discounts, payments to employees, and referral services. The two areas of primary interest to most ophthalmologists, however, are routine waiver of Medicare co-payments and investment in small business entities. The rules on the former provide that the routine waiver of co-payment and deductible amounts is not protected unless the patient is eligible for Medicaid or one of the other similar federal assistance programs for indigent individuals.

The rules for investment are more complex. Investments in large, publicly traded companies with assets in excess of $50 million are usually protected. Investments in smaller entities are more stringently regulated and must meet all eight of the standards outlined below:

1. No more than 40% of the value of investment interests can be held by those in a position to make or influence referrals or generate business for the entity.
2. The terms offered to a passive investor in a position to make referrals can be no different from those offered to other passive investors.
3. The terms offered a passive investor who is in a position to make referrals must not be related to the expected volume of referrals.
4. There can be no requirement that an investor make referrals as a condition to remaining an investor.
5. The entity must not furnish any items or services differently to passive investors than to noninvestors.
6. No more than 40% of the gross revenue of the entity may come from referrals or services generated by investors.
7. The entity cannot loan or guarantee funds for an investor if the funds are used to invest in the entity.
8. The return to the investor must be proportional to the investment interest held, and not to the amount of referrals generated.

Investors who invest in smaller, physician-owned entities will have a very hard time meeting all of the above standards, especially numbers 1 and 6. In fact, these provisions will effectively remove almost all physician-owned operations from protection under the safe-harbor regulations. In particular, free-standing optical shops that are not a part of the ophthalmology

---

Figure 4.6. The 11 Safe Harbor Areas

1. Investments
2. Space rental
3. Equipment rental
4. Personal services
5. Sale of medical practice
6. Referral services
7. Warranties
8. Discounts
9. Payments to bona fide employees
10. Group purchasing
11. Routine waiver of Medicare co-payments

Adapted from American Medical News, August 12, 1991, p. 33.

practice and surgery centers will be in jeopardy. It is important to realize that this will not necessarily make the operation fraudulent or illegal. It simply means that it will not be automatically protected in the event that it is investigated by a federal or state agency, and that the entity may need to show that the business practices are neither fraudulent nor abusive. In many instances this may prove to be both time consuming and expensive.

Compliance can be achieved if the optical shops and other similar businesses are made a part of the ophthalmologist's practice rather than a separately incorporated entity. Problems can also be avoided by simply not doing business with Medicare-eligible individuals. It is likely that additional safe-harbor situations may be proposed in the future, and it is hoped that optical shops and free-standing surgery centers will be among them. It is important for ophthalmologists with interests in this area to follow closely additional legislative developments, and to consult with their attorneys for additional advice.

Why the fraud and abuse statutes anyway? The issue arose because of the concern that doctors, by referring patients to entities in which they have an ownership interest, unnecessarily increase health care costs. Physicians, writing in both the popular[19] and medical literature,[20-22] deplore the perception of the crass commercialization of medicine that these arrangements evoke.

A study performed in Florida indicates that at least 40% of physicians who are involved in direct patient care have an investment interest in a health care business to which they could refer. Nearly half hold interests in diagnostic imaging centers.[23]

There is also increasing evidence to indicate that physicians who have an ownership interest in a business tend to utilize that service more frequently than those who have no such financial arrangement.[24-27] Although this increased usage is not necessarily inappropriate, the possibility that it may be has attracted the attention of Congress and the press.

The problem has been addressed by the AMA in a somewhat confusing fashion. The Council on Ethical and Judicial Affairs, supporting the position adopted by the Board of Directors in 1991, declared in May of 1992 that, in general, "physicians should not refer patients to a healthcare facility outside their office practice at which they do not directly provide care when they have an investment interest in the facility,"[28] unless they can demonstrate that there are no alternative facilities or financing arrangements available. However, in June of 1992 the House of Delegates reversed this position and declared that self referral was ethical as long as the patient is fully informed about the arrangement. At a subsequent meeting in December, however, the House of Delegates again adopted the position that self referral was not ethical unless there was a clear-cut community need. No one knows for sure what tomorrow will bring.

Representative Fortney "Pete" Stark, a major sponsor of the original Fraud and Abuse legislation, introduced even more restrictive legislation in 1993. This bill, known as the "Comprehensive Physician Ownership and Referral Act of 1993," would prohibit referrals from physicians to any entity in which they have an investment interest, whether the source of payment is public or private.[29] At present, the regulations apply to Medicare patients only. The services that would be forbidden are listed in Figure 4.7.

Leasing companies are more than willing to provide a line of credit for ophthalmology practices. A leasing company will provide the desired equipment by buying it and then renting (leasing) it to the practice for a specified period of time. In theory, someone who leases equipment pays only for the use of the equipment rather than the expense of outright ownership of an item whose value begins to depreciate as soon as it is acquired.

Leasing usually provides the advantage of a low initial outlay (e.g., no down payment or sales tax are required) and a regular monthly payment, which is tax deductible and is frequently lower than that needed for outright purchase. Protection against ownership of obsolete equipment is built in because title to the equipment is retained by the leasing company and it can be returned at the end of the lease if desired. In addition, the use of a lease keeps the credit line of the practice available for additional borrowing.

Purchase of equipment allows development of an equity position. This means that when the equipment is paid for, the practice will own something of value. The value, however, will usually be less than the price paid because of depreciation—the reduction of value of an item that occurs because of wear and tear, obsolescence, and various other considerations. Some ophthalmologic equipment (e.g., slit-lamps, chairs, stands) retains its value well. Other equipment, particularly high-technology items such as lasers, computers, and certain mechanized cataract removal systems, becomes worth much less as soon as the "new improved model" is released. This often seems to occur within minutes of the purchase of the current model.

Unlike a lease payment, a loan payment used to purchase equipment cannot be deducted in its entirety each month for tax purposes. A depreciation schedule must be assigned for each piece of equipment, and only that amount, plus interest costs, can be deducted.

Whether leasing or buying equipment ends up being the most economical choice can be a complicated matter that depends on how each transaction is structured and on the type of equipment involved. The lease must be carefully prepared to ensure that it is not construed as an installment sale contract. It should be carefully evaluated to see who is responsible for additional

LEASING VERSUS BUYING

Figure 4.7. Comprehensive Physician Ownership and Referral Act 1993, Restricted Services

Clinical laboratory services	Parental and parenteral nutrition equipment and supplies
Physician therapy services	Outpatient prescription drugs (pharmacies)
Occupational therapy services	Ambulances
Radiology services—including magnetic resonance imaging, computed tomography, and ultrasound	Home infusion therapy
Durable medical equipment	Inpatient and outpatient hospital services

Source: American Medical News, January 25, 1993, p. 3.

costs such as personal property tax, maintenance, and insurance. The purchase price of the equipment (if purchase is desired) at the end of the lease period must be understood and factored in. Many banks will tailor a purchase transaction to resemble a lease, thus decreasing the monthly outlay. An experienced accountant should be able to evaluate these (as well as any additional) factors for each situation to determine the best structure for the transaction.

OFFICE SPACE LEASE CONSIDERATIONS

All lease arrangements for the practice should be reviewed by the attorney before they are signed. It is important to remember that everything in a lease is potentially negotiable and that it never hurts to ask for changes to be made. In the terminology of the lease, you are the lessee and the other party is the lessor.

Prospective sites should be evaluated for location, tenant mix, condition of the property, and possible zoning restrictions, and the satisfaction level of the current tenants should be probed. Adequacy of public restroom and other facilities, and access to the building during nonbusiness hours, should be considered. Sufficient and convenient parking for both patients and staff is essential.

It is usually much less expensive to build in unfinished space than it is to remodel. If substantial remodeling is required, the plans should be made an addendum to the lease agreement and initialed by both parties. The division of responsibility for construction planning, execution, and expenses should be made clear, and rent should not commence until the space is available and functional for business use. A penalty clause requiring financial compensation for late or substandard construction may help to ensure timely completion.

All lease agreements must contain certain information, including the initial term of the lease, rental rate (usually per square foot), and options for subsequent renewal. The right of first refusal on adjacent space is essential. This means that you should be given the first opportunity to acquire additional contiguous office space before it is offered to another physician. In addition, the contract should specifically identify which party is obligated to pay for maintenance expenses in common areas, utilities, insurance, real estate, and personal property taxes.

If possible, an escape or cancellation provision should be included in the event the physician dies or becomes totally disabled and unable to practice. If this is not possible, a sublease option giving the physician the right to re-rent the space to another individual is essential. Escalator clauses giving the lessor the right to pass on increases in utilities and other expenses to the lessee are usually included and are not necessarily unreasonable. The index chosen as the guideline should be related to the cost of leasing property (and not the price of eggs in Budapest), and a maximal figure above which the rent cannot be raised must be clearly specified.

Most leases indicate that fixtures attached to walls or floors become a part of the space and cannot be removed. If you are planning expensive cabinetry or wall coverings that you may want to keep if you relocate, be sure that provisions for this are included in the lease agreement. In addition, some leases require restoration of the space to its original condition at the end of the lease term. This can sometimes be very expensive, and this stipulation should be avoided if possible.

The choice of location and the layout of a medical office are important factors in developing a successful ophthalmology practice. Assuming that an option is available and that you are not simply joining an established practice, the office location should be selected to minimize travel between home, office, and hospital. It is important, however, that the office be developed in an area of true need rather than in an area that is merely convenient.

The office should be easily accessible to patients by both automobile and public transportation. Parking facilities must be both adequate and convenient for patients and staff; handicapped access must be available. Medical buildings are popular because their location is often well known to patients, they have the requisite handicapped facilities and suitable electrical and plumbing capacities, and other physicians are available to provide both referrals and consultative services. They also tend to have ancillary services, such as pharmacies and optical shops, available. However, lease rates are often high, and cleaning and maintenance services may be substandard.

Many hospitals are making attractive offers to young physicians in an effort to develop long-lasting relationships. They provide interest-free or low-interest loans to help with start-up costs, office space in hospital-owned buildings at reduced rents, and assistance in obtaining necessary equipment. This is done with the hope of encouraging admissions to the hospital and use of other hospital facilities, such as laboratories and outpatient surgical centers. Because certain financial incentives and arrangements may conflict with Medicare fraud and abuse regulations, all contractual agreements should be carefully reviewed by legal counsel before they are finalized.

Free-standing (excluding surgi center) and strip center medical office space are rarely used by ophthalmologists in larger urban areas. The concern is that they are isolated from other medical professionals and may convey a "cheap" appearance to patients. This is not the case in more rural areas, where converted small homes are often used. Except for very unusual situations, the medical office should not be located in the home of the physician.

OFFICE LOCATION

One of the most important considerations in developing plans for an office is its size. The most serious error that can be made is to make the initial office too small. The additional monthly rent spent to ensure an adequate size, even if some space is initially left unused, is small compared with the cost of moving an office because the current space has been outgrown. A minimum of 1,200 square feet should be obtained for a single practitioner, and 1,500 square feet is not excessive. Those planning for additional services on premises (e.g., dispensing, orthoptics, office operating room) should increase the size accordingly.

All offices should provide for a separate private entry for the physician that bypasses the waiting room. The waiting room itself should allow 16 to 20 square feet for each patient, and sufficient chairs should be provided for the family members that often accompany them. A space that seats 12 to 14 individuals is usually enough for a single ophthalmologist who sees up to 6 patients per hour. If space permits, a separate section for children will be appreciated by young and old alike. A no-smoking policy for the waiting room should be mandatory.

The chairs in the waiting room should be individual, with straight backs and arms for comfort and to facilitate rising and sitting. Benches, couches, and linked chairs should be avoided because patients will go to great lengths (including standing) to avoid sitting next to someone they do

OFFICE PLANNING

not know. Magazines should be current and varied in content, and large-print items provided if possible. Incandescent rather than fluorescent lighting provides a warmer, more inviting appearance.

Carpeting of the waiting area, halls, and business area, and wall coverings rather than paint, reduce noise and decrease maintenance expenses. Appropriate background music may be appreciated by the patients, but the system should provide for shut-off switches in examination rooms. Halls and doorways should be wide enough to accommodate walkers, wheelchairs, and stretchers.

A separate dilating room or alcove is useful to improve patient flow. This avoids tying up an examination room while waiting for a patient to dilate, and movement from one area to another gives the patient the sense that some progress is being made. It is best not to dilate patients (especially children) in the waiting room because the reaction may frighten other children who may not need the drops. Lighting should be subdued for comfort, and reading materials provided for use until the patient's vision becomes too blurred.

Individual examination rooms can use either mirrors or a "long lane." It is wise to have at least one long lane if it is anticipated that children will be seen, because once the children spot the mirror behind them they will usually not cooperate by looking straight ahead. An animated toy or TV cartoon system at the far end of a long lane is also helpful when children are to be examined.

A minimal room width of 8 feet is needed for comfort and easy use of examining equipment. Several additional chairs are needed to accommodate family members. In most instances, at least two rooms should be available to allow better patient flow. They should be similarly equipped so that the examiner is equally comfortable in both. Coat hooks should be provided in the rooms (even if they are also available in the waiting or common areas), because patients are often reluctant to leave possessions behind. Additional rooms for services such as patient education, visual fields, and contact lens fitting also help to encourage smooth patient flow.

The secretarial and business areas must be large enough to allow efficient operation. This area is the one that is most frequently made too small. Good lighting and comfortable chairs and desks are essential, and adequate numbers of telephones and other business necessities are mandatory. Waiting to borrow the only adding machine available is not an efficient use of employee time.

Computers (discussed in more detail separately) are becoming increasingly common for both billing and word processing chores, and sufficient desk space, power, and wiring are essential. A fax machine and a high-quality copier are important time-savers. The office manager should have a separate area that is relatively private to allow discussions with patients concerning financial and other sensitive information. A separate staff lounge for breaks and lunch is another nice touch.

Office overhead is a major drain on the income of a practice. Every dollar spent is one less dollar available to be taken home in your paycheck. New practitioners, fresh from training programs in which every conceivable piece of equipment is available, often try to duplicate that situation in their own offices. Each piece of equipment desired should be evaluated to determine if it is really essential for proper patient or fiscal management. Fancy equipment that looks nice but fails to generate enough revenue to pay for itself should be avoided.

PRACTICE CASH FLOW MANAGEMENT

BILLING AND COLLECTING

To be successful, all businesses must handle their financial transactions carefully. The guidelines for a medical practice are no different from those for any other business. Three important factors must be considered:

1. Collect funds as promptly as possible.
2. Keep the funds in your possession as long as possible.
3. Maximize the return on the funds while they are in your possession.

An essential consideration for any business is the ability to collect promptly the monies owed it. Medical practices are no exceptions to this, and there is no need to apologize for or feel uncomfortable about being paid for services rendered. A capably run practice actually helps to contain medical costs by keeping overhead expenses as low as possible, reducing the necessity for frequent fee increases.

Essential to any billing and collection effort is accurate biographic data on each patient. Patient information forms that facilitate gathering this information are commercially available or can be developed, if needed, for each individual practice. Patients are often quite mobile, and the information should be updated regularly. Without an accurate address, phone number, and place of employment, collection attempts may be impossible.

Payment at the time office services are rendered is the least expensive and most efficient method of collection. In most instances this is also convenient for patients, if they have been informed in advance that this is the policy of the practice. In particular, patients without insurance coverage, emergency patients, and those who may be difficult to find in the future should be asked to pay at the time of service. Exceptions to this rule can be made when appropriate, but frequent deviations will undermine the purpose of the policy. It is important for the physician to be committed to the policy, to convey this commitment to everyone involved in the process, and to provide suitable training for staff members before asking them to perform this function. Any charges not paid become part of the accounts receivable of the practice.

All patients should be given an itemized bill (frequently referred to as a *superbill*) at the end of the visit, with the total charge calculated. This document should contain the proper ICD-9 diagnosis and CPT service codes so that it can be easily submitted by the patient to the insurance carrier. If payment is not made at the time of service, the patient should be asked to assign payment of all insurance proceeds directly to the physician. Usually there is a place on the superbill or insurance form where the patients sign to do this, preventing them from receiving the payment and keeping it.

If a portion (but not all) of the bill will be paid by an insurance company, it is especially important to collect all applicable co-payments and deductibles when services are rendered, because the cost of billing for these small sums is prohibitive. Prompt receipt of payment for products dispensed (e.g., contact lenses, glasses, and drugs) is also important, as significant expenses to the practice are often associated with providing these items. Failure to receive payment under these circumstances results in an actual net cash loss for the practice.

Although some physicians regard payment of professional charges by credit card as "too commercial" and "not professional," more and more practices are utilizing this method. It is convenient for patients and obviates excuses such as "I left my checkbook at home" or "I don't have the money with me." The funds become available for immediate use (the credit card receipts are deposited to the practice bank account just like a check), and the cost for the service (usually 3% to 6%) is small and may actually be less than the cost of billing. Local or state medical societies often have special arrangements with banking institutions to provide credit card services at reasonable cost. In addition, some banks may be willing to reduce their charges in return for a formal business or personal banking arrangement.

A patient who does not pay at the time of the office visit should be given an itemized statement as a bill, along with a preaddressed return envelope. If the payment is not remitted promptly, a second statement requesting payment should be sent with a return envelope. Additional follow-up billing for slow payers should be prompt; the longer the charge remains open, the less likely it is to be collected. It is therefore important to be able to follow closely the age of the accounts receivable owed to the practice. Various systems available to assist in this process are discussed below.

For patients who cannot pay the charges in full, a payment plan should be established and the patient's adherence to the schedule carefully monitored. Interest charges are not usually collected, but when they are it is essential to comply with federal and state truth-in-lending laws. Collection agencies, if required, should be professional, responsible, and experienced in medical collection techniques. There are strict rules regarding the methods that collection agencies can use, and the practice may be held liable for the errors of the agency it hires.

Physicians have a longstanding tradition of providing care for patients regardless of their ability to pay, and billing and collection procedures for medical practices should take into account the financial situation of the individual patient. Compassion should be an important consideration in all collection decisions. No patient should be denied needed care because of an unpaid balance. In addition to the ethical problems involved, such action may subject the physician to the serious charge of patient abandonment.

Although patients with typical indemnity insurance coverage are ultimately responsible for all charges, many wait until they receive payment from their insurance company before paying the physician. Therefore, insurance carriers are a significant source of revenue for most ophthalmic practices, and efficient billing techniques are critical for prompt payment. The Academy has recently published the Insurance TPR (Third Party Reference) which provides many practical suggestions for dealing with Medicare and other carriers.

The most important item necessary to ensure prompt payment is accurate coverage data for each individual patient. This information, including carrier name, relevant policy numbers, responsible party, and billing address, should be updated each time the patient is seen to avoid needless payment delays caused by billing the wrong carrier. When possible, a list should be maintained for each insurance company detailing whether or not payment for routine eye exams is a benefit, so that a claim will not be submitted for uncovered services.

Billing of insurance carriers should be done promptly. In particular, surgical charges that involve large sums of money should usually be submitted within 48 hours after the procedure. Insurance companies tend to postpone payment as long as possible for almost any reason (so that they can continue to earn interest on the funds), and physician-induced delays only exacerbate the problem. When available, use of electronic billing systems (see below) can speed reimbursement and minimize the chances that an insurance company employee will delay the claim.

Payment of claims pending from each company should be tracked closely, and those not promptly received should be actively followed and the charge resubmitted if necessary. Be certain that the information sent to the carrier initially is complete and correct (a "clean claim"), because delays will otherwise be inevitable. If possible, try to establish a personal relationship with an individual in the claims or professional services department of the companies with which you deal frequently. This person, if treated properly, may be invaluable in helping you to solve payment problems.

DEALING WITH INSURANCE CARRIERS

Dealing with managed care systems presents many varied and unique problems. Primary among these is that patients are no longer ultimately responsible for payment for medical services. Instead, a formal contractual arrangement for payment between a third party and the physican is substituted and physicians become vendors of services, to be dealt with by these companies just like any other vendor.

As noted in Chapters 2 and 4, the percentage of practice income derived from the various forms of managed care systems currently in place has been rising and will probably continue to rise as more and more employers make this option the one most financially attractive for employees to choose. Because patient-paid premiums, co-payments, and deductibles are usually lower in managed care systems than in more traditional plans, employees (especially those at the lower end of the wage scale) are being be forced by economic considerations to choose these restrictive systems without fully understanding all of the consequences.

Managed care contracting for ophthalmology services can run the gamut from an ophthalmology directed primary care program to provision of specialized tertiary services.[1] In the former system, ophthalmologists direct the delivery of all eye care services, with supervised optometrists commonly providing many of the primary services. This strategy lends itself to

MANAGED CARE SYSTEMS
GENERAL COMMENTS

either a capitated payment system (the mechanics of which are defined below) or discounted fee-for-service, and protects patient access to ophthalmologists, which may be a problem when optometrists or primary care physicians function as gatekeepers. Outside of an HMO (Health Maintenance Organizatiom) model, development of this type of plan can present significant administrative hurdles as ophthalmologists struggle to either provide or direct a primary care network.

Groups of ophthalmologists who are involved in providing secondary eye care services to a large number of patients under a managed care contract run a significant financial risk if the program is not adequately managed and financed. Fees are almost always lower than those obtained under traditional indemnity plans, and the administrative work involved may be both burdensome and costly. Because most ophthalmologists have limited experience in this area, it is important that adequate professional advice be obtained before any such contracts are signed.

Development of regional tertiary care delivery systems to provide specialized or highly sophisticated procedures for large groups of patients (patterned on the "centers of excellence" concept used for delivery of cardiac and transplant services) is another form of managed care. Such centers can see a large enough number of patients to develop cost-effectiveness and outcome data for high-technology procedures, and can therefore compete on the basis of quality rather than merely cost. The contracts often are either discounted fee-for-service or based on a global payment to the medical center that covers both physician and hospital charges. Unfortunately, these programs may interfere with established referral patterns, and may also provide insufficient income to fund the traditional research and educational activities normally associated with academic centers.

Whether or not an ophthalmologist participates in a managed care plan depends to a large extent on the specific situation in the community. In many areas where the penetration of these groups is small, avoidance is still possible. In most areas, however, the percentage of patients who belong to managed care systems is increasing, and it is becoming increasingly difficult for practices to remain outside the system.

There are potential benefits from participating in managed care contracts. For example, the patient base for the practice can be increased. In addition, these patients can refer friends and relatives (who may not be members of managed care plans) and often purchase noncovered services such as glasses, contact lenses, cosmetic services, and pharmaceuticals. The plans can provide a relatively steady cash flow and, for practices that are not completely booked, can fill empty patient slots at very little increased cost. Many of the patients will remain loyal and stay with the practice even if their insurance coverage changes.

There may be significant disadvantages as well. The lower reimbursement provided by these plans means that the same work is being done for less money. In addition, the administrative burdens add costs not normally encountered in fee-for-service arrangements, thus reducing the net income of the practice even further. The patients' loyalty to the practice may be largely coverage driven and may therefore vanish with alteration of provider agreements. It may become difficult to see patients because of strict gatekeepers who are forced to refer them first to optometrists, and some plans make consultations difficult to obtain even when medically indicated. According to a recent survey in *The Physician's Advisory*,[2] HMO and PPO (Preferred Provider Organization) payments to ophthalmologists, on average, approach 72% of the full fee-for-service amount. Almost 90% of those reporting indicated that the payment they received was approximately equal to or greater than their Medicare/Medicaid fees. Average payment time for fee-for-service payment was 42.3 days after billing, with surgeons waiting about 1 week longer for receipt of funds.

Contracting with managed care companies is an extremely complicated endeavor. A detailed checklist of the items to be considered is shown in Figure 5.1. Therefore, advice from accountants, actuaries, attorneys, and practice management consultants with experience in this area is essential. Although a comprehensive review of this subject is beyond the scope of the present chapter, several important considerations are discussed below.

SPECIFIC MANAGED CARE CONTRACTING CONSIDERATIONS

Of primary importance is the solvency and reputation of the plan with which you are dealing. It is vital to know who is actually responsible for payment (e.g., employer, insurance company). The market position in the community of the plan being evaluated should be investigated, as well as its financial stability and viability. Review the membership data distributed by the company and obtain independent verification of the numbers if possible. Determine whether or not the projections for market penetration promised by the plan have been achieved, and whether the patients to be added to the practice will be new ones or merely old patients converted to a managed care product. Plans that cannot deliver a volume of patients sufficient to overcome the reduced fees offered should be avoided. Learn the identity of the executives of the plan and analyze their record in the industry. Investigate the plan's record on payment of claims, financial reserves, and distribution of withholds and other financial incentives. At all costs, avoid allowing a single managed care vendor to constitute too high an overall percentage of the practice volume.[3,4]

PLAN ASSESSMENT

It is most important to understand exactly how you will be paid for services rendered. Most HMOs and PPOs pay a discounted fee-for-service and may even withhold a portion of the fee, which will be remitted only if certain conditions are met. Because most withholds are never returned, they should be subtracted from the fee before calculating the discount given to the managed care group. For example, a service for which $100 is charged under fee-for-service, and $80 with a 10% withhold under a managed care system, would be an actual fee discount of 28% rather than 20% ($80 - $8 = $72/$100 = 72%).

FINANCIAL ANALYSIS

Capitation (payment based on a certain dollar amount per HMO member per month) can be profitable if calculated properly and a disaster if it is not, because it is difficult to be certain exactly what type of patients will be assigned to the practice and what level of services will be required. Although actuarial advice may be necessary to determine precisely the rate needed to be the equivalent of a fee-for-service billing, a rough calculation can be made by picking a subpopulation within your own practice that matches the demographics of the HMO in question, and calculating the average amount billed per individual during the calendar year. Be sure to include the costs of related ancillary services for which you may actually be responsible under a capitated contract, and revenues from co-payments and any fees paid for noncapitated services. This number then becomes the standard to which the actual capitation rate is compared.[5]

Figure 5.1. Managed Care Contracting: Checklist Considerations

PARTIES
- Clearly identified.
- Correct contracting entity.
- All parties with obligations pursuant to the contract are included.
- Date contract signed/effective.

PREFACE
- Recitals consistent with terms of contract.
- Recitals do not contain additional representations or obligations not found in body of contract.

DEFINITIONS
- Clearly defined terms.
- Defined terms capitalized throughout contract.
- Consistent use of terms throughout contract.
- Definitions of covered and non-covered services.

TERM
- Effective date of contract.
- Procedure and notice period for renewals, if any; generally avoid automatic renewals.

TERMINATION
- Termination with and without cause.
- Remedy period for termination with cause.
- Notice requirements.
- Rights and duties upon termination.
- Right to compensation at usual and customary charges after termination.
- Survival of important terms after termination, e.g., confidentiality, indemnification, medical records, etc.
- Impact of termination in event that plan takes unilateral action which is not acceptable to physician.

PHYSICIAN'S DUTIES
- Scope of services provided (full range or only specific services).
- Consistent with qualifications/specialty.
- Exclude ethically objectionable services.

- Right to refuse to treat disorderly/problematic patients.
- Verification of eligibility procedure.
- Pre-admission certification procedure.
- Professional and general liability insurance requirements.
- Prior approval for specified services.
- Patient referral limitations (adequate base or referral providers).
- Indemnification scope and ramifications (note that endorsement to professional liability insurance should be requested to cover any indemnification obligations). Avoid indemnification for independent actions of plan.

PLAN'S DUTIES
- Plan's obligation to compensate physician clearly spelled out.
- State certifications, if appropriate.
- Verification of eligibility procedure.
- Pre-admission certification procedure defined.
- Coordination of benefits.
- Grievance procedure.
- Marketing (use of physician name controlled).
- Professional and general liability insurance and indemnification requirements.
- Does the plan provide security (e.g., deposit agreement in the event plan does not process/ pay claims in accordance with contract).
- Avoid limitations on plan's responsibilities for care or outcomes.

UTILIZATION REVIEW
- Duties and costs clearly defined.
- Types of review defined: pre-admission, concurrent, retrospective.
- Specific standards for UR determinations.
- Appeal procedure.
- UR procedure incorporated into contract.

PHYSICIAN COMPENSATION
- Physician's right to bill members for copayments, deductibles, and

noncovered services.
- Methodology for renegotiating rates clearly defined.
- Time limitations on claims submission.
- Claims turnaround time acceptable.
- Penalty for failure to pay claims in agreed time frame.
—Charge interest on unpaid balance.
—Revert to paying billed charges.
- Billing form.
- Interim billing.
- Avoid any attempt by plan to coordinate fees under agreement with fees under other agreements (most favored nations clauses).

MEDICAL RECORDS
- Maintain as required by law.
- Plan obtains written patient authorization for release of records.
- Plan pays copy costs.
- Access by plan in accordance with law and subject to applicable confidentiality requirements.

GENERAL PROVISIONS
- All attachments included and incorporated into contract.
- Amendment.
- Arbitration and costs.
- Assignment.
- Attorney's fees.
- Binding effect.
- Choice of law.
- Compliance with terms.
- Confidential information.
- Entire agreement.
- Exclusivity on either party.
- Grievance procedure (HMO especially).
- Identifications of other contract providers.
- No agreements with other providers regarding prices.
- No blank spaces.
- Notices.
- Provisions separable.
- Rights of members.
- Rights of parties.
- Section headings.
- Signature block.
- Unforeseen circumstances.
- Waiver of breach.

Prepared for the St. Louis Metropolitan Medical Society by Mark Goran, Partner, Sonnenschein Nath & Rosenthal, August 1992. Reproduced by permission.

Be certain that the capitation payment is calculated as an actual amount and not as a percentage either of the premium charged or of the amount actually collected from the payer. If the percentage method is used, an HMO that wants to gain market share may lower its premium, and consequently your income will go down. If only the collected payments are considered and the HMO happens to be inefficient or the payer goes bankrupt, you will bear the burden.

A recent review in *Argus*[6] pointed out that although many physicians have a natural aversion to the concept of capitated medical care (since it is based on the premise of the less care delivered to the patient, the higher potential profit for the doctor), such care can have several financial advantages for many practices. Prepayment for services rendered enhances cash flow, with no wait for claims to be submitted, reviewed, denied, resubmitted, re-reviewed, finally paid, eventually mailed, and at long last posted. Billing and collection costs are virtually eliminated and bad debts are also reduced. Capitation rates may approach 80% of the fee-for-service reimbursement, which is higher in many instances than the discounted fee-for-service payments offered by the companion PPO. This rate of reimbursement, when coupled with the reduced administrative costs noted above, may make a capitated system attractive to more practices in the future.

Group size and composition are very important in assessing risk. Plans with a large number of members under 2 years or over 65 years of age may show increased utilization of services. Groups of less than 20,000 non-Medicare lives may be difficult to rate actuarially and can expose the physician to significant financial risk. Purchase of outlier insurance for protection from adverse patient selection in capitated groups can help to lower the burden.

Terminology is very important when capitated plans are evaluated. For instance, payment per *member* per month is very different from payment per *subscriber* per month. In the former, each individual insured life contributes to the capitation reimbursement. Under the subscriber definition, each *family* is considered to be the billing unit, so that physicians are paid the same for a single individual as for a family of four. Carefully investigate all of the payment definitions before you sign the contract.

Regardless of the compensation mechanism involved, it is essential that the practice develop accurate cost data for the services delivered. This information may not be readily available in the standard format used by most practices to track expenses, which breaks them down into broad categories such as salary, supplies, and rent. True cost accounting involves the allocation of the appropriate portion of both fixed and variable practice expenses to given procedures and services. If this information is not available, rates of payment may be accepted that will not cover the actual cost to the practice of providing the service and the practice will actually *lose money* on each service provided.[7] Losing money on each case and "making it up on volume" is not a profitable way to run an office!

In addition to the actual rates of payment involved, administrative considerations are also significant. It is important to evaluate the timeliness of payments under both capitation and discounted fee-for-service, as well as the overhead costs of collecting and tracking the payments. Onerous regulations can easily devour the administrative savings generated by capitated payments. If possible, capitated payments should be due and payable on the first day of the month, with financial penalties for delays of more than 5 days. Fee-for-service payments should have a window for billing of at least 90 days, with provisions for rebilling without penalty for claims "lost" by the agency. In addition, payments should be received within 30 days, with interest accruing after this time period.

Payment schedules offered by managed care systems should be compared both with standard fee-for-service reimbursement and with each other. Managed care systems offering terms that are distinctly out of line should be approached about extending more favorable rates; otherwise, consideration should be given to terminating the relationship with the plan.[2] The leverage that physicians have in negotiating better financial terms in a contract is directly proportional to the value of the physician or physician group to the plan. Plans that need to expand their provider base to increase market penetration will be forced to offer more attractive rates. Conversely, well-established plans often have control over a large segment of the patient population and may be able to attract physicians at lower reimbursement rates in return for the promise of increased patient volume. Provisions for regular rate increases should be built into all contracts, with the inflation adjustment linked to a recognized index such as the CPI.[8]

Point-of-service plans are hybrid HMO–PPO products that enable the patient to decide at the time services are rendered whether or not to remain within the provider network or to seek care from an outside physician. These plans usually impose a significant financial penalty on patients who go outside the provider panel, with co-payments and deductibles approaching 30% to 40% of charges versus the 90% to 100% coverage provided for care received from the approved providers. It is important that network physicians not be financially at risk for the costs of out-of-network care that exceeds the plan budget. Since patients can self-refer and there is no effective utilization review of the outside physicians, it is possible for patients to receive unnecessary expensive treatments over which plan physicians have no control. Out-of-plan providers may also entice patients with the promise of waiver of co-payments and deductibles. A strong physician panel is the best protection against large numbers of patients seeking care outside the system.[9]

"HOLD-HARMLESS" PROVISIONS

Hold-harmless clauses[10] in managed care contracts are inserted to shift responsibility for economic liability from the plan back to the physician members. These clauses state, directly or indirectly, that the physician will indemnify (i.e., protect) the plan from loss, damages, or costs (including attorneys' fees) arising from any acts committed by the physician. The desire on the part of managed care plans to include these clauses in the contracts has arisen from the recent assessment of damages against managed care companies for actions by non-employee physicians. The liability assumed by agreeing to these clauses is *not* covered by standard medical malpractice policies, as insurance companies are unwilling to assume the risk of underwriting such an open-ended proposition, which can be construed to include such items as libel, slander, contract default, interest, and loss of profits.

These clauses take many forms, including some that may seem innocuous on the surface because they do not contain the words "hold-harmless" or "indemnify." Phrases such as "agree to assume all risks" and "this is a release from" are actually hold-harmless clauses in disguise. So are warranties that quality of care will meet community standards or that physicians are solely responsible for all treatment decisions (even if they are forced into making certain decisions because of utilization review policies of the managed care organization).

Before they are signed all managed care contracts should be reviewed by experienced health law attorneys who will look for both obvious and less explicit indemnification language. In addition, it may be useful to try to include a specific clause to the effect that "neither party shall be responsible for any liability of the other party, unless such responsibility is expressly assumed."[3] When possible, both parties should be required by the contract to secure and retain separate malpractice insurance policies with limits sufficient to protect their individual interests. This ensures that the plan will remain solvent even if it loses a malpractice judgment. If mutual indemnification clauses are required, each party "should purchase insurance that names both parties and protects each from claims of bodily injury, death, or property damage arising from the activities of the physician or other party or their respective agents, servants or employees associated with the contract."[8]

PLAN DEFINITIONS AND TERMINATION PROCEDURES

All contracts have a portion that deals with definitions. These sections, which are often ignored by physicians, are important! They define such critical concepts as "emergency," "specialists," "quality assurance," "covered service," and "medical necessity." They also define risk pools, capitation rates, service areas, and other critical concepts. This section must be read and understood before the contract is signed.

It is important to understand how long the contract runs and how it can be amended and/or terminated. Most contracts run on a calendar year basis and are automatically renewed if notice of termination from the physician is not received 90 days in advance. The document usually specifies that the contract can be terminated for cause by the managed care company if the physician loses the right to practice medicine, cannot obtain malpractice insurance, is convicted of a felony, or is guilty of gross misconduct. Similarly, the physician can terminate the agreement if the plan declares bankruptcy or fails to make appropriate payments. In particular, nonpayment of fees should permit termination of the plan contract with 30 days' notice, and the post-termination obligations of the physician should extend for only a brief period thereafter. Open-ended agreements that obligate the physician for an indeterminate period of time (i.e., until "the plan can make appropriate arrangements for the transfer of patients to another provider") should be avoided, as a bankrupt plan may have significant difficulty in recruiting new physicians to care for its patients.[6] Be sure that the plan cannot unilaterally amend the contract by simply notifying the physicians in writing. Utilization review and quality assurance requirements should also be defined in the contract, and the terms and conditions carefully reviewed. Participants should understand who will be doing the reviews, what the grievance procedures are for both patients and physicians who disagree with the findings, and whether or not arbitration is available as a mechanism for resolution of disputes. How physicians will be initially credentialed for acceptance into the plan and subsequently for continuation should be defined, and an appeals procedure for denials outlined. The administrative structure of the plan must also be investigated. Are referrals needed for all visits? Who is responsible for obtaining them? Is the mechanism cumbersome for verifying the eligibility of individuals to be treated? Can retrospective denials be used to force physicians to return funds they have already collected (and probably spent?)

If at all possible, no "by reference" items should be included. These are documents referred to in the contract but not actually a part of it. In effect, participating physicians are being asked to agree to provisions that they have not had the opportunity to review. Many of these noncontract items can be modified unilaterally by the managed care company, and such changes can alter the contract significantly. Be sure you have the chance to review, comment on, and modify these provisions, and the freedom to terminate your contract with the plan if material changes have been unilaterally inserted.

ACCOUNTS PAYABLE MANAGEMENT

Once the money due is actually collected, the practice must also have a mechanism for paying its bills (called accounts payable) and handling any excess cash on hand. Proper handling of the large sums of money that pass through a medical practice can significantly contribute to the bottom line without much additional effort on the part of the physician. Your accountant or management advisor should be consulted for assistance in this area.

Conscientious efforts should be made to minimize balances in non-interest-bearing accounts (such as checking accounts) and to keep as much money as possible in money market and other short-term instruments. Because bank "money market" accounts often pay rates well below those of standard money market mutual funds, you should investigate carefully. Since bills are usually paid in groups, money can be transferred as needed into the checking account when checks must be written. For large account balances, banks may be willing to "sweep" money automatically from the checking account into one paying interest and to transfer funds automatically back into the checking account as checks are cleared. Compare the interest rates and charges for the checking account and all other services to find the most economical arrangement.

Many vendors complain that physicians are poor payers when it comes to meeting their own practice obligations. Your accounts payable should be settled in timely fashion but not necessarily as soon as the bills are received. Look for the due dates and make payments by that time. Look for discounts on the invoices and be sure to take them if payment is made on schedule. Ask for additional discounts for large or bulk purchases or when payment is made at the time of delivery.

Credit cards can also be used to purchase items and defer payment. If you use cards that do not charge interest when the outstanding balance is paid in full each month, you obtain in effect an interest-free loan for about 45 days. Consequently, if several cards are available with different billing cycle cut-off dates, the proper card can be chosen to extend the payment due date as far into the future as possible.

COMPUTERS IN MEDICAL PRACTICE

As in many other areas, improvements in computer technology and decreasing hardware costs have contributed to the increasing dependence on computers in medical practices. It is now possible to interface with university and hospital mainframes, literature search systems and other educational services, insurance carriers, investment houses, and other individuals with equipment that is easy to use, reliable, and financially within the range of most physicians.

In addition to the uses mentioned above, other practical applications are helpful in the day-to-day operation of the practice. Therefore, it seems essential to have some sort of computer capability in the office from the very beginning of practice. Although the IBM® PC or one of the IBM clones is the most common type used, the Apple® Macintosh® is increasing in popularity because of its ease of use. Programs are also now available that allow transfer of information between these two systems.

One of the most important uses of a computer in the office is word processing. Preparation of letters to referring physicians, hospital order forms, patient instruction sheets, and other materials is much easier with word processing program than with a typewriter. Because the computer and a letter-quality printer make it easy to revise materials and reprint them, there is a lesser tendency to settle for something that is not quite right. Laser printers, although slower than good dot-matrix printers, produce documents that are difficult to distinguish from those prepared by a professional printing service. Desktop publishing programs enable in-office creation of patient newsletters and other educational materials custom-tailored to the individual practice.

Another important use of computers is electronic transmission of insurance claims. This is easily done with a modem (basically, a telephone connection device) and software that is frequently provided by the carrier. It is not necessary to have a completely computerized office to take advantage of this special capability, which is included in most commercially available office management packages.

The primary advantages of using this form of communication with the insurance company are speed and accuracy. The information goes directly from your computer to the one in the office of the insurance carrier. No time is lost in mailing paper claims to the company and having an insurance company employee re-enter the data. In addition, there is less likelihood for loss and mislaying of claims, with resultant delay in reimbursement. Unless the claim is unusual, there is no manual review of electronically submitted claims, which also speeds payments.

A third important use of computers is financial management. It is impossible to run an ophthalmic practice efficiently without access to accurate and timely data on overall practice performance. Availability of income and expense information and the ability to compare it easily to data from previous years are critical in guiding decisions regarding practice management and development. This type of information is also available from the practice accountant, but it is nice to have it available on-line.

Again, it is not necessary to have a totally computerized office to take advantage of this tool. Many financial management programs are available. One very simple system, Quicken®* (Intuit, Menlo Park, Ca.), is extremely easy to use, very inexpensive, and very powerful. It can write and print checks, track expenses by category, balance the checkbook, prepare payroll if desired, and easily generate a number of very useful business reports, including cash flow and profit-and-loss statements. It has password protection at two levels to prevent unauthorized access and alterations, backs up easily, and is probably all that many offices will need.

The principal defects of Quicken® are the absence of an audit trail (no individual passwords or operator numbers for each user are presently available) and the ability to alter transactions without preservation of the original entry. In addition, the double-entry bookkeeping and depreciation schedules desired by some accountants are not easily accomplished. Although these deficiencies are potentially troublesome, the overall package remains quite attractive.

One additional important use of computers is in the area of integrated office management: patient billing, scheduling, and medical records. This is what physicians are describing when they say they "are computerized." These systems, using single or multiple linked units (a network), can manage almost all essential office tasks. Most are modular in concept, allowing initial pur-

INTEGRATED OFFICE MANAGEMENT SYSTEMS

chase of only those capabilities thought necessary. For example, an office could start with only patient billing and add scheduling later if needed.

In the past, the cost of these systems was often prohibitive for new practitioners. Now that the packages are becoming much more affordable, the advantages of starting practice with an integrated system should be considered. This is particularly true for physicians whose ultimate goal is to have such capacity in the future and for those who deal extensively with managed care systems that have stringent fee schedules and billing requirements. Physicians who are interested in keeping track of specific diagnoses and/or treatment plans will also find a computer system extremely useful.

A reasonable starting package should include, at a minimum, a single station with a 486-33 mHz or equivalent processor, adequate RAM and hard disk capacity, and a near-letter-quality dot-matrix printer. The system should be expandable (a system without networking capacity should not be considered) and should be able to generate patient statements, to age accounts receivable, to track insurance company balances, to print insurance forms and patient mailing labels, and should have some electronic billing capabilities. Integrated word processing capability and accounts payable systems add additional flexibility. When not connected to the system, each computer can function alone and can be used for any normal computer application. An excellent review and comparison of the various systems currently available was recently published.[11]

Once the decision has been made to obtain this type of computer system, the choice of vendor is the next consideration. Making the incorrect decision will cause both immediate and long-term problems. Start by investigating the vendor to find out how long the company has been in business, the number of systems in place, and the number of ophthalmologists using the system. Talk with individual system users and with friends and colleagues to identify the good and bad points of the systems available. Obtain information concerning the following critical areas:

1. Ease of use and operation ("user-friendly").
2. Reliability of hardware and software.
3. Training and installation procedures.
4. Ongoing support capabilities (e.g., costs, availability).
5. Ongoing operating costs.
6. Upgrade and expansion capabilities.
7. Adequate financial analysis capabilities and audit safeguards.

It is also important for you and your office staff to actually try the system hands-on, and to compare the various options for ease of operation. Look at the instruction manuals to see if they are clearly written and contain useful and relevant information. Be certain that any contract signed includes complete pricing information, performance standards, appropriate penalties for nonperformance, and installation deadlines. Try to make a single vendor responsible for both hardware and software to prevent system incompatibilities and "turf battles" over which component is at fault if there is a breakdown. Most important is that the software source code (the information that is the "brains" of the system) be placed in escrow so that, if the vendor goes out of business, the program can be made available to another vendor to permit continued operation of the system.

It is also possible to have computer billing capability without actually having a system in house. There are companies that will prepare computer-generated statements from paper systems used in your office and delivered to them by mail or courier service. Some can also do third-party billing electronically. One problem with such a system is that it first demands creation of paper records and requires two manipulations of the same data to complete processing.

Another strategy utilizes in-office "dumb" terminals (those without stand-alone computer capability) that connect via phone lines to a central processing unit that is used by many different practices. In such a system, the advantages of single entry of information and the speed of on-line transmission of data are preserved, and the computer company simply provides statements, insurance forms, and electronic billing using the data entered directly from your office. However, these systems are somewhat inflexible, in that your office billing cycle must conform to the schedule set by the vendor. In addition, because the computer terminals are "dumb," they have no word processing or other computer capabilities.

Good billing systems are also available for practices that choose not to use computers. The best of these is generically referred to as a "pegboard" system. It uses numbered superbills, individual patient ledger cards, and a day sheet on which all transactions are posted. Charges are posted on the superbill, ledger card, and day sheet simultaneously, ensuring that all contain the same information. Billing is done by photocopying the ledger card and sending the copy as a statement to the patient or responsible party.

The pegboard system is simple, relatively inexpensive, and generates a patient statement immediately. There are built-in safeguards to ensure that payments are posted and that accounts remain in balance. This system works reasonably well in a relatively small office without multiple third-party payer contracts.

The disadvantages of this type of system include the difficulty in aging accounts receivable, problems with keeping track of third party payer accounts and managed care system balances, and inability to easily analyze individual diagnoses and patient demographic characteristics. It is possible to age the accounts receivable in this system by attaching different-colored clips to the individual ledger cards as they are copied, with each color representing a certain age, but this is both time consuming and labor intensive because the cards must then be pulled and the data compiled manually. In addition, the financial integrity of the system requires the total of the ledger card to equal the account balance listed on the day sheets. This means that the ledger cards must be totaled frequently or the process becomes subject to both honest errors and the possibility of embezzlement. Practices that use this system must be disciplined enough to perform this function regularly, a task frequently neglected by many offices.

To bill and collect properly for services rendered, it is necessary to use the coding systems required by insurance carriers when they process claims. With increasing frequency, carriers are demanding that diseases and services be identified with these systems rather than narrative descriptions, even when paper claims are submitted. With rare exceptions, when electronic billing is used only the coding systems are accepted.

OTHER BILLING
OPTIONS

PEGBOARD SYSTEMS

**CPT AND ICD-9-CM
CODING**

There are two major components of the system: service codes (CPT) and diagnosis codes (ICD-9-CM). The former are used to describe the type of service the patient received and the latter to indicate the condition for which the services were provided. Many physicians delegate the choice of these codes to the billing and insurance personnel on their office staff. In most instances this is unwise because the staff may not be familiar with all procedures that are performed. Incorrect coding can result in either underpayment and loss of income or overpayment with subsequent exposure to charges of fraud and abuse. All physicians should have a working knowledge of both the CPT and ICD-9 systems, as well as an understanding of specific local carrier policies applicable to services and procedures commonly performed in their own practices.

For a well-written and more comprehensive discussion of the coding systems and how to use them, both *The Guide* (see the annotated bibliography section on practice management after this chapter) and *Managing Your Medical Practice* have excellent sections. Several professional ophthalmology organizations (including the Academy) also sponsor seminars on coding that are well researched and presented. These are especially useful because they deal only with the aspects pertinent to ophthalmologists.

As mentioned earlier, most practices use a form of superbill to keep track of charges. These usually have commonly performed services and procedures printed on them (complete with the CPT code) as well as a list of diagnoses (with ICD-9 codes). Therefore, it is necessary only to circle the appropriate items and forward the slip to the billing staff. It is best for the physician to designate the proper choices rather than leaving this task to a clerk, who may omit charges while reviewing the chart. In the long run, time is actually saved and billing performed more promptly and accurately.

CPT CODING

The term *CPT* is short for Current Procedural Terminology. The system used was developed (and copyrighted) by the AMA and is periodically reviewed and updated. Each specialty organization (including the AAO) has input in this process. Nevertheless, new services and procedures often do not have appropriate codes, which may cause problems.

Because the system is revised yearly, proper reimbursement demands use of the current volume. Be sure to have sufficient numbers of copies available for all who need them. There are also "minivolumes" available for ophthalmology, which are much less bulky and easier to use than the larger books. Each volume has an introductory section that explains in detail how the system works and offers many examples. This portion of the text should be read by both physicians and their staff so that all have a clear understanding of how CPT codes work.

The federal government also has a system called *HCPCS*. This system (the Health Care Financing and Administration Current Procedural Coding System) includes the CPT codes as its primary component. In addition, there are Level 2 codes to provide additional information about certain specific areas, and Level 3 codes (currently being phased out) that allow local carriers freedom to create additional codes and modifiers as needed. Current copies can be obtained through the local Medicare carrier.

In general, the CPT system is complete but also complex. There are specific codes for various services and a series of modifiers that can be added to explain and define each item in more detail. These suffix modifiers enable additional information about each service to be communicated in a standardized fashion. A detailed discussion of the various modifiers and their proper use is contained in the introductory section of the CPT handbook.

Certain codes are "global" (they include various individual services grouped together), whereas others are not. When a global code is available for a given service (such as a comprehensive eye exam), it should be used rather than billing separately for the individual components of the exam. Similarly, the code for cataract extraction with lens implant (66984) includes performance of an iridectomy as an integral part of the procedure. Billing for the iridectomy in addition to the cataract procedure would be an example of "unbundling," and is illegal.

The CPT system designates certain other services with an asterisk (*) adjacent to the CPT code number. Some of the starred procedures commonly used in ophthalmology include removal of a foreign body, corneal scraping, epilation for trichiasis, and lacrimal probing. Formerly the asterisk indicated that the code included the procedure only and that any additional services necessary (such as pre- and postoperative care) could be billed for separately. This may still be true for private carriers, but for Medicare patients the rules have changed. Most of these procedures now include a 10-day postoperative global period during which no additional charges related to the procedure are allowed. Be sure to mark the superbill so that these codes are distinguished from major surgical procedures, in which the longer 90-day postoperative global period applies.

The CPT codes used to report evaluation and management (E/M) services for office visits, in-patient and outpatient consultations, hospital care, confirmatory consultations, and emergency department services were completely changed in 1992.[12] Several key concepts recur throughout all of the codes. They include the extent of the history, level of examination, complexity of medical decision making, counseling services offered, and time spent in direct contact with the patient. Each code level (1–5) is clearly defined by a combination of the various factors outlined above. For example, a low-level new patient office visit (99201) involves a problem-focused history and examination with straightforward medical decision making. The highest level new patient office visit (99205), on the other hand, would consist of a comprehensive history and examination, as well as medical decision making of considerable complexity. The time involved at the lowest level would average 10 min in direct patient contact, in contrast to 60 min for the highest-level service.

Time is a particular concern for ophthalmologists who make extensive use of technical personnel, because face-to-face time spent with patients is often shortened in such circumstances. Both the AMA and HCFA stress that the times are averages, not to be used strictly by carriers in determining reimbursement levels. HCFA emphasizes that time is merely a secondary factor by stating that "the typical times shown in the visit code definitions are not, and have never been intended to be, the defining factor in how to code a visit. We will undertake training and educational activities with Medicare carriers to ensure that this is fully understood."[13]

Because the new coding system is so complex, the level of service code chosen should be supported by documentation in the medical record. Some examples of vignettes along with the approved CPT designation are shown in Fig. 5.2. The Academy has proposed modifications to the documentation guidelines for the E/M system codes in an attempt to make them more understandable and less arbitrary, and it is hoped many of the suggestions will be accepted for use in 1994.

In 1993 (and probably in 1994), ophthalmologists also have the option of using the old 92000 series to code intermediate and comprehensive examinations for old and new patients. The disadvantage of using these codes is that they are not all considered as primary care codes (the new codes are), and therefore payments will not be automatically increased if reimbursements for all primary care codes are raised. In addition, new physicians who use the 99000 series do not have their reimbursement decreased by 20% because the new physician reduction does not apply to codes designated as primary care codes.

The correct use of office codes is essential to obtain proper reimbursement. Various levels of service are provided, depending on the specific needs of the patient at each encounter. All patients do not need, and should not undergo, a comprehensive examination each time they are seen in the office. Therefore, it is important for the office to use the variety of codes available for various clinical situations.

As a general rule, the higher the level of service, the greater the payment. It is essential that the code used correspond to the level of service actually delivered and that the level be the correct one for the diagnosis listed. The details of the examination performed should be carefully documented in the chart, so that questions raised later by third-party payers regarding levels of service can be properly answered. For example, a diagnosis of acute conjunctivitis does not usually justify a comprehensive eye examination. In fact, the CPT manual uses the diagnosis and initiation of treatment for acute conjunctivitis as an example of a less extensive examination. A physician using the higher code could be accused of "upcoding" in an attempt to obtain increased reimbursement and might therefore be required to return the excess payment. A pattern of upcoding can expose the physician to the serious charge of insurance fraud. If, because of unusual circumstances, a higher than normal level of service was required, the physician should outline the reasons for it and document the extent of these additional services in the patient record.

There are also special codes for certain special ophthalmic services, such as visual fields, fluorescein angiography, gonioscopy, and extended fundoscopy. Carriers are sometimes inconsistent in their treatment of these codes, especially with regard to bilaterality. For example, does the code for gonioscopy cover one eye or both eyes for billing purposes? Each private payer should be contacted and asked about its specific policy for the following commonly used codes:

92020: gonioscopy.
92081–83: visual fields.
92225–26: extended ophthalmoscopy, initial and follow-up.
92285: external ocular photography.
90100: serial tonometry.
92120: tonography.
92140: provocative tests for glaucoma.
76515–19: A-scan.

However, for Medicare patients, the new RBRVS regulations specifically state that a diagnostic service performed only on one eye requires the use of a reduced service modifier along with the code.

REFRACTION

The policy for reimbursement for refraction is particularly confusing. Most carriers consider refractive services to be an integral part of a comprehensive examination. They include the measurement and prescription of corrective lenses as part of the examination fee and do not allow a separate charge to be made. Medicare, however, does not follow this policy. It considers determination of the refractive state to be an "uncovered service" and will not pay for it. Consequently, refraction is not subject to any charge limitations, a separate additional fee can be established, and the patient can be asked to pay on both assigned and nonassigned claims.

It was formerly necessary to indicate whether or not a refraction was performed during the examination and treatment of Medicare patients. Under the new rules, however, HCFA will not consider refraction to be a part of any examination, because it is not a covered service and was not measured

---

Figure 5.2. AMA-Validated Clinical Examples

99201: Initial office visit for a 10-year-old girl for determination of visual acuity as part of a summer camp physical (does not include determination of refractive error).

99203: Initial office visit for a 55-year-old female with chronic blepharitis. There is a history of use of many medications.
Initial office visit for an 18-year-old female with a 2-day history of acute conjunctivitis. Extensive history of possible exposures, prior normal ocular history, and medication use is obtained.

99205: Initial office visit for a 29-year-old female with acute orbital congestion, eyelid retraction, and bilateral visual loss from optic neuropathy.
Initial office visit for a 70-year-old diabetic patient with progressive visual field loss, advanced optic disc cupping, and neovascularization of retina.

99213: Subsequent office visit for a 65-year-old female, established patient, with primary glaucoma for interval determination of intraocular pressure and possible adjustment of medication.

99214: Subsequent office visit for a 68-year-old male, established patient, with the sudden onset of multiple flashes and floaters in the right eye due to a posterior vitreous detachment.

99221: Hospital admission for a 12-year-old with a laceration of the upper eyelid involving the lid margin and superior canaliculus, admitted before surgery for IV antibiotic therapy.

99223: Initial hospital visit for a 71-year-old patient with a red painful eye 4 days following uncomplicated cataract surgery due to endophthalmitis.

99244: Initial office consultation for a 28-year-old male, HIV positive, with a recent change in visual acuity.
Initial office consultation for a 45-year-old myopic patient with a 1-week history of floaters and a partial retinal detachment.

99245: Initial office consultation for a 67-year-old male with a negative past ophthalmic history is referred with a 3-day history of a red painful eye with blurred vision due to acute angle-closure glaucoma. The patient is dehydrated from nausea and vomiting.

99254: Initial hospital consultation for a 43-year-old female for evaluation of sudden painful visual loss, optic neuritis, and episodic paresthesia.

99262: Follow-up inpatient consultation with 45-year-old male, established patient for discussion of CT scan which demonstrates a cavernous hemangioma.

99282: Emergency department visit for a young adult patient with injected sclera and purulent discharge from both eyes without pain, visual disturbance, or history of foreign body in either eye.

99283: Emergency department visit for a patient who has a complaint of acute pain associated with a subjected foreign body in the painful eye.

during the Hsiao study. If a refraction is performed, it is usually submitted as a separate and distinct item (CPT for 1992 designates 92015 as the correct code), with its own charge. It will not, however, be paid by Medicare.

ICD-9-CM

The ICD-9-CM system* for indicating services rendered is even more complex than the CPT codes discussed above. In addition to providing a comprehensive mechanism for documenting disease processes, it also includes codes for symptoms, signs, and ill-defined conditions: congenital abnormalities, injury and poisoning, and various other miscellaneous classifications. Each code has three to five digits, depending on desired and required specificity. Certain codes are allowed by insurance companies for billing purposes, whereas others are rejected for reasons that are not always clear. Punctuation is important, as is the order in which codes are listed. Medicare and most other insurance carriers now require these codes to be used for billing purposes in place of narrative descriptions.

There are also special color-coded editions of the code book to assist in determining the diagnosis codes that are generally accepted by the insurance carriers. Codes that usually work are coded in green, questionable ones appear in yellow, and those usually not accepted are indicated in red. This information is helpful in avoiding reimbursement delays due to improper coding. The Academy recently has published a very useful, inexpensive ophthalmology booklet, *ICD-9 Ophthalmology,* which is much easier to use than the longer volume.

The coordination of CPT and ICD-9 coding is extremely important. It is necessary that service codes (CPT) be linked with appropriate diagnosis codes (ICD-9) to obtain proper compensation and avoid charges of performing unnecessary procedures. For example, use of the service code for trabeculectomy (66170) with the diagnosis code for senile nuclear sclerotic cataract (366.16) is inappropriate because the procedure is not indicated for the treatment of cataract. Such a claim would probably be rejected by the insurance company. Use of the proper diagnosis code (primary open-angle glaucoma, 365.11) will correct the problem.

Technically, the ICD-9 code used should be the one that best describes the reason why the patient came for the visit, not the diagnosis made during the examination. According to the rules, if additional problems are detected their presence will not justify altering the original diagnosis code or increasing the level of service at that examination. As an example, if a patient comes in because of a red eye (found to be acute conjunctivitis) and glaucoma is also discovered, the level of service should remain at that corresponding to the original diagnosis, regardless of the supplementary tests that may have been performed. To obtain proper reimbursement, the patient must be told that another problem has been discovered and asked to return for the additional tests required.

When several diagnoses are present at the time of the visit (such as cataract and glaucoma) and when services are needed and provided for each, every procedure performed should be specifically linked with the proper diagnosis code. This can be done either by submitting individual claims for each diagnosis and appropriate service(s) or by designating the correct ser-

---

*The complete manual is available from: ICD-9-CM, P.O. Box 971, Ann Arbor, MI 48106; (313) 769-1597. Its introductory section provides detailed instructions on the correct use of the system.

vice/diagnosis pairing in the space provided on the claim form. Leaving this process to chance and/or the discretion of the insurance carrier usually results in delayed or inadequate payment.

Some carriers, in an effort to reduce payments to physicians, have begun to include separate and distinct services as part of a global diagnosis code. For example, some are declaring that gonioscopy and extended fundoscopy are part of a comprehensive ophthalmologic examination, even though it has been customary to regard them as separate procedures. The carriers then disallow payment for the additional services, even when there is no question of their appropriateness. Such arbitrary determinations on the part of the carriers should be appealed to the medical director of the company. Experience indicates that they have been reversed in many instances.

Carriers (Medicare in particular) may also limit the number and kinds of visits that will be covered within a given time period. They may cover only one comprehensive visit per calendar year and disallow any others, even when medically indicated. For example, consider the case of a patient who has had a comprehensive examination for evaluation of a cataract and then presents 2 months later with painful diplopia. A second comprehensive examination may be required to evaluate the new condition properly, but the carrier may reject the claim even though the diagnosis is different, because the patient has already had a comprehensive exam. Sometimes the carrier will allow the claim but reduce it to an intermediate examination ("downcoding"). When such situations occur, it is necessary to file an appeal with the carrier and to provide any additional documentation needed to support the claim.

Medicare patients must be informed in advance if it is probable that a service will not be covered. If there is a question, patients should be informed of this possibility and asked to sign a waiver (the "medically unnecessary letter") stating that they will accept financial responsibility for the charges if payment is denied by Medicare. If they are not given this information and the payment is ultimately denied, neither the patient nor Medicare can be asked to pay for the service (even if it was medically necessary). The physician simply ends up working for free.

Such situations are likely to occur when multiple office visits are needed within a relatively short period of time. Patients with active uveitis or those with poorly controlled glaucoma typically encounter this problem. In addition to protecting themselves by having the patient sign the waiver described above, physicians should vigorously protest these inappropriate denials of proper medical treatment, even though they usually involve relatively small amounts of money; not to do so simply allows further intrusion by non physicians into the doctor–patient relationship.

PAYMENT APPEALS

All insurance carriers have mechanisms that enable patients and physicians to appeal reimbursement decisions. These mechanisms are different for each carrier, and the procedures required must be followed to the letter if there is to be any chance of overruling a previous decision. The medical record, operative report, and any other available information that might be useful to support the appeal should be submitted to justify the request for reconsideration. Careless and incomplete records virtually guarantee that no additional compensation will be forthcoming.

Medicare has a particularly cumbersome system for appealing denials and downcoding problems. Either the patient or the physician can initiate the appeal. Despite the work involved, physicians should protest (or assist the patient in doing so) when they feel that denied or reduced services were medically necessary or when they believe that the allowed amounts for covered services were incorrect. All necessary documentation in support of the appeal should be sent to the carrier along with the "Request for Review of Part B Medicare Claim" form (available from the carrier).

When the carrier review process proves unsatisfactory, it is possible to obtain a "hearing" from the carrier. This process, which can take place in person if desired, provides a second opportunity to convince a different individual that the claim is valid. The amount involved must be greater than $100, but claims reviewed and denied within the preceding 6 months can be pooled to reach that amount. If this process is unsuccessful, the physician or beneficiary still believes that the determination is in error, and the amount in question is more than $500, a third appeal can be undertaken before an Administrative Law Judge of the Social Security Administration. The request for this hearing must be filed within 60 days of the carrier's adverse decision. A further appeal of amounts in excess of $1,000 is available through judicial review.

MEDICARE FRAUD AND ABUSE

Physicians who are notified that they are being charged under the provisions of the Medicare Fraud and Abuse Act should take this communication very seriously. They should promptly attend to all requests for information and should obtain advice from an attorney and/or malpractice management consultant with experience in dealing with this problem.

MEDICARE PARTICIPATION VERSUS NONPARTICIPATION

The decision of whether or not to become a participating physician is based on many factors, and not solely on economics. These factors include personal preference, local custom, and patient demands. It is important, however, to understand the financial consequences of each option before a decision is made. Participating physicians agree to take assignment on *all* claims for *all* patients for a defined period of time, usually 1 year. This means that they will accept as payment in full the Medicare Fee Schedule amount, with 80% of this amount received directly from Medicare and 20% from the patient.

Nonparticipating physicians can selectively take assignments for individual patients or services. The patient is responsible for payment of the entire charge and the portion paid by Medicare is sent directly to the patient. For 1993, the charge that nonparticipating physicians can make for a service is limited to 115% of the Medicare Fee Schedule amount (the *limiting charge*). Because the MFS allowable payment for nonparticipating physicians is only 95% of that for those who participate, the increased reimbursement for nonparticipators is actually only 109.25% of the value for those who participate (115% x 0.95.= 109.25%).

Whether or not a nonparticipating physician is better off financially participating depends on the actual percentage of claims that are accepted on an assigned basis. At the extremes, if *no* claims are accepted and all fees are collected, nonparticipating physicians will earn 9.25% more than if they had participated. If *all* claims were accepted they would earn only 95% of what they could have been paid. For most physicians, the truth is obviously somewhere in between.

As a general rule, if more than 65% of the charges (*not* claims) are processed on an assigned basis, the physician is better off participating (Fig. 5.3). As the collection rate decreases from 100%, the actual break-even percentage is even lower. For those purists who would like to calculate their percentage more precisely, the formula is shown below (assuming that the collection rate on assigned claims is 100% and that there are no collection costs for unassigned claims):

$$100 = 0.95\,x + y\,[1.0925\,(100 - x)]$$

where x = percent assigned claims, $100 - x$ = unassigned claims, and y = collection percentage on nonassigned claims.

Obviously, physicians should have in place a mechanism for determining the percentage of charges that are submitted on an assigned basis if they are to make use of this type of analysis. Computer billing systems can often provide this information. If none is available, an approximation based on a study of 2 or 3 months of charges may prove helpful. Some of the other advantages and disadvantages are outlined in Fig. 5.4.

Although Medicare is the primary insurer for most patients over the age of 65, in some cases it is not, and failure to bill the proper primary carrier will lead to delays in reimbursement.[14] If patients (and their spouses) over age 65 are employed and have benefits payable under an Employer Group Health Plan (EGHP), the employer plan becomes the primary insurer. Patients do have the option of declining this coverage, in which case Medicare again becomes the primary insurer. In this instance, however, the employer-sponsored coverage cannot be used as a secondary insurer.

When Medicare is the secondary carrier, the Medicare Fee Schedule limits do not apply and the normal office charges can be used. The amount received from the primary insurer must be accepted as payment in full, and no money can be accepted from the Medicare beneficiary. If the EGHP declines to pay for the service and it is a covered service under the Medicare program, then Medicare must pay.

MEDICARE AS SECONDARY PAYER

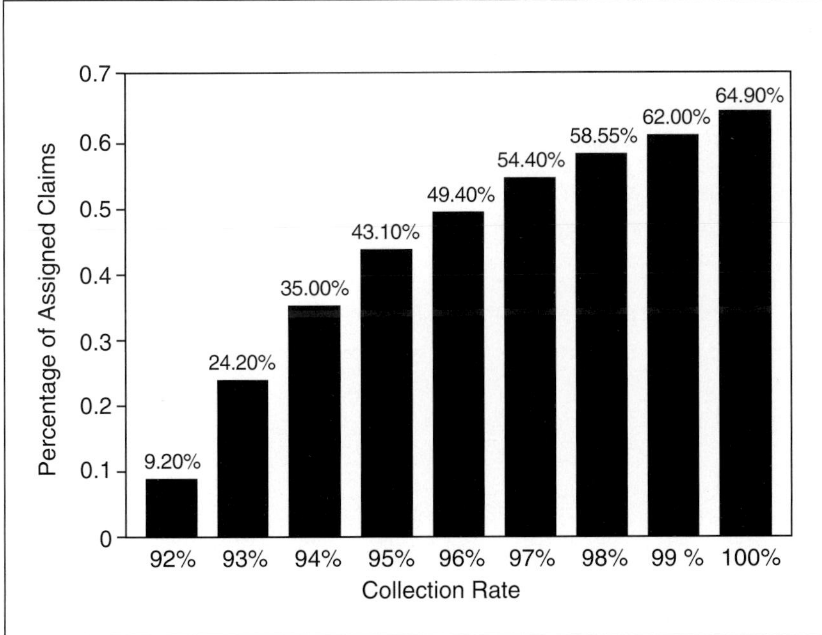

5.35 | Medicare breakeven analysis, 1993, for nonparticipating physicians. Greater assignment rates result in revenue less than participating physicians receive at the same collection rate.

The rules for disabled individuals are also complicated. For those incapacitated with end-stage renal disease, federal retirees, and employees of small businesses, Medicare remains the primary carrier. For employees under age 65 and their spouses, Medicare becomes secondary to the large group health-plan insurance provided by the employer. Therefore, it is important that the employment status of all disabled Medicare-eligible patients be verified to allow proper billing.

Medicare is the secondary payer for medical expenses incurred as a result of an automobile accident, regardless of who was at fault, and the primary auto insurance carrier must be billed first, even when the policy seems

---

Figure 5.4. Pros and Cons of Medicare Participation

ADVANTAGES OF PARTICIPATION
1. Ability to raise customary charges.
2. Higher prevailing (5%).
3. No need to maintain a separate Medicare charge schedule.
4. Faster payment on clean claims (21 days vs. 26 days).
5. Exempt from financial disclosure requirements on *elective* procedures over $500.
6. Collection effort for reimbursement centers on insurers not patients.
7. Referrals from Medicare.

ADVANTAGES OF NONPARTICIPATION
1. Preserves patient/physician relationship.
2. Can collect up to the full limiting charge from patient.
3. Limiting charge is higher than prevailing charge allowing increased revenues.
4. Can collect payment reductions such as Gramm–Rudman.

DISADVANTAGES OF PARTICIPATION
1. Limited to collection of deductibles and coinsurance from secondary payers.

DISADVANTAGES OF NONPARTICIPATION
1. Pressure to maintain dual charge schedule unless all patients are charged the limiting charge.
2. Financial disclosure requirement on elective procedures over $500.
3. Slower Medicare payment to beneficiary delaying collection.
4. EOMB (Explanation of Medical Benefits) message to patient emphasizes increased cost of nonparticipating physician.

Adapted by permission from Third Party Reimbursement (TPR) Insurance.

to indicate otherwise. If the insurer pays part (but not all) of the charge, Medicare can be billed for the remainder. If the insurer pays the charge in full, Medicare has no further responsibilities. Similarly, if patients have a claim against a liability insurance carrier, Medicare should not be billed until the claims against that carrier have been exhausted. In addition, Medicare should not be billed for expenses that would typically be covered under Workers' Compensation plans.

To help identify patients for whom Medicare is the secondary carrier, the following questions should be asked of all Medicare patients:

1. Do you or your spouse work for a company that provides group health insurance?
2. Is the treatment related to an automobile accident?
3. Is the treatment related to an accident or injury at work?
4. Is the patient eligible for Veterans Administration benefits?
5. Is the patient covered by the United Mine Workers or is a retired railroad employee?

RETIREMENT PLANNING

This topic should be an important consideration for all physicians from the time they enter practice. Physicians in academic medicine or in other salaried positions, such as HMOs, may have future retirement provided for as part of their employment contract. Those hired as employees in a private practice setting may or may not have such benefits available, depending on the particular situation. Physicians who start practice on their own should consider this area as carefully as they do all others. Even if a decision is made not to fund a program immediately, it is important to have a definite program in mind that can be implemented as the practice develops.

Many types of retirement plans are available, but the rules that govern establishment of and eligibility for the various options, as well as the tax consequences involved, are constantly being changed. Therefore, professional advice should be sought from other physicians, attorneys, practice management consultants, and other professionals with experience in this area. *Future Focus* (see Recommended Readings) has a well-written section on financial planning for residents and new practitioners and can serve as a starting point for obtaining information in this area. *The Guide* also has a section that can be consulted. The most important thing is to begin to "think retirement" from the first day of practice; this will make it much easier to provide for the future.

It is hoped that the following data will give some idea of how funds accumulate, the value of compound interest, and the effects of inflation on the need for a given level of income. Figure 5.5 shows how much money will be available after a given period of years if $100 is invested at the beginning of each month at various rates of return.

The effect of inflation on retirement income needs is shown in Figure 5.6. According to this table, a physician who feels that retirement would be comfortable at a present salary level of $50,000 would need $132,500 in 20 years, based on an annual inflation rate of 5% ($50,000 × 2.65).

Finally, Figure 5.7 indicates how long accumulated funds will last at various rates of investment income and withdrawal of original capital. This brief introduction should emphasize the complexity of planning for retirement and the need to address these concerns promptly on entering practice.

Figure 5.5. Growth of Funds at Various Rates of Return

YEAR	5.5%	7%	8%	9%	10%	12%
1	1,236	1,246	1,253	1,260	1,267	1,281
2	2,542	2,583	2,611	2,638	2,667	2,724
3	3,922	4,016	4,061	4,146	4,213	4,351
4	5,380	5,553	5,673	5,795	5,921	6,183
5	6,920	7,201	7,397	7,599	7,808	8,249
6	8,546	8,968	9,264	9,572	9,893	10,576
7	10,265	10,863	11,286	11,730	12,196	13,196
8	12,080	12,895	13,476	14,091	14,740	16,153
9	13,996	15,073	15,848	16,672	17,550	19,482
10	16,024	17,409	18,417	19,497	20,655	23,234
15	28,002	31,881	34,835	38,124	41,792	50,458
20	43,762	52,397	59,295	67,290	76,570	99,915
25	64,496	81,480	95,737	112,953	133,789	189,764
30	91,780	122,709	150,030	184,447	227,933	352,991

This table shows how much you have at the end of a period of years if you save or invest $100 a month, assuming various annual returns. Other amounts can be calculated as fractions or multiples of $100. (Table assumes $100 is saved at the beginning of each month.) Adapted from *The Wall Street Journal*, Dec. 6, 1989.

Figure 5.6. Inflation Factor Table

No. of Years Until Retirement	Rate of Inflation						
	3%	4%	5%	6%	7%	8%	9%
5	1.16	1.22	1.28	1.34	1.40	1.47	1.54
8	1.27	1.37	1.48	1.60	1.72	1.85	1.99
10	1.34	1.48	1.63	1.79	1.97	2.16	2.37
12	1.43	1.60	1.80	2.01	2.25	2.52	2.81
15	1.56	1.80	2.08	2.40	2.76	3.17	3.64
20	1.81	2.19	2.65	3.21	3.87	4.66	5.60
25	2.09	2.67	3.39	4.29	5.43	6.85	8.62

The income that will provide a comfortable lifestyle in your first year of retirement will be eroded by inflation as the years go by. To find out how much money you will need in future years, multiply your first year's retirement income (or the current year's income, if you are already retired) by the appropriate inflation factor in this table. For example: If your current annual income is $35,000 and you want to know how much annual income you will need in 15 years if inflation remains at about 5%, multiply $35,000 by 2.1. The answer: $73,500. Adapted from *Investment Vision*, Fidelity Investments.

Figure 5.7. How Long Will the Money Last?

Account Growth Rate	Original Capital Withdrawal Rate										
	6%	7%	8%	9%	10%	11%	12%	13%	14%	15%	16%
12%	—	—	—	—	—	—	—	22	17	14	12
11%	—	—	—	—	—	—	23	17	14	12	11
10%	—	—	—	—	—	25	18	15	13	11	10
9%	—	—	—	—	26	20	16	14	12	11	9
8%	—	—	—	28	20	16	14	12	11	9	9
7%	—	—	30	22	17	14	12	11	10	9	8
6%	—	33	23	18	15	13	11	10	9	8	8
5%	36	25	20	16	14	12	11	9	9	8	7

Before you start drawing on investments in retirement, a little advance planning may be required to ensure that the money will last as long as you do. The table shows, for example, that if the value of your retirement account grows at a rate of 6% a year and you are taking out 15% of your original capital each year, the money will last 8 years. Cut your withdrawals to 10% and the money will not run out for 15 years. You can also use the table to gear your withdrawals to how long you want the money to last. Suppose you decide assets must last 15 years and you estimate that they will grow at an annual rate of 10%. In that case, the table shows that you can withdraw roughly 13% of the value of your original capital each year. A dash means that at that rate of withdrawal, the money will never be exhausted.

ADDENDUM

Since this book was written, several important events have taken place. The Omnibus Budget Reconciliation Act of 1993 (OBRA '93) was passed by one vote in both the House and Senate and signed by the President. This bill promises a reduction in the deficit of $500 billion over the next 5 years, including savings of $56 billion from the projected growth of the Medicare program. Even with this cutback, expendures of the Medicare program are still expected to rise to $239 billion by 1998, almost double the level in 1992.

Ophthalmology was not hurt as much as initially feared. In fact, it is estimated that the reimbursement for major ophthalmologic procedures will actually increase by about 2% in 1994. Medicare payment updates for 1994 have been fixed at 8.6% for surgical services, 6.6% for primary care, and 4% for other services. Although self-referral regulations were toughened in many areas, glasses and contact lenses remain exempt when dispensed as an integral part of the ophthalmic office practice.

In a major victory, the policy of reduced Medicare payments to new practitioners (discussed in Chapters 2, 4, and 5) was changed after a concerted effort by all of organized medicine. Starting in 1994, all physicians will be compensated at the same rate, which should enhance the value of a new associate to an established practice, and increase income for those who choose to practice solo.

REFERENCES

1. Council on Ethical and Judicial Affairs of the American Medical Association: *Current Opinions.* Chicago: American Medical Association, vii-ix.
2. Beauchamp GR, Bettman JW, Stromberg CD: *Ethics in Ophthalmology: A Practical Guide.* San Francisco: American Academy of Ophthalmology, 1986.
3. Dyer AR: Ethics, advertising, and the definition of a profession. *J Med Ethics 1985;11:72–78.*
4. Pellegrino ED: What is a profession? The ethical implications of the FTC order and some Supreme Court decisions. *Surv Ophthalmol 1984;29:221–225.*
5. *Ophthalmology Times* May 1, 1991, 6.
6. *The Guide: A Handbook to Building and Maintaining a Successful Ophthalmologic Practice.* San Francisco: American Academy of Ophthalmology, 1991.
7. Margo CE: Advertising in ophthalmology. I. A threat to professional autonomy. *Surv Opthalmol 1988;33:211–214.*
8. Spivey B: *Statement of the American Academy of Ophthalmology to the Subcommittee on Health, House Ways and Means Committee.* San Francisco: American Academy of Ophthalmology, Jun 14, 1990.
9. Magano M: *Statement for the Subcommittee on Health, House Ways and Means Committee on Medicare Fraud, Waste and Abuse.* Washington, DC: Government Printing Office, Jun 14, 1990.
10. Saunders DR: Analysis of the OIG study, "Outpatient Surgery: Medical Necessity and Quality of Care." *Ocular Surgery News* Feb 1, 1991, 32.

1. Foreman J: National health care spending: Where do the dollars go? *Arch Ophthalmol 1993;111:34.*
2. Ginsburg JA, Prout DM: Access to health care. *Ann Intern Med 1990;112:641–661.*
3. Health care: A magic asterisk? *The Wall Street Journal* Jan 25, 1993, A1.
4. Berk ML, Monheit AC: The concentration of health expenditures: An update. *Health AFF (Millwood) 1992;11(4):145–149.*
5. Health and Medical Services: US Industrial Outlook 1993. United States Department of Commerce, Jan 1993, 42–44.
6. Borzo G: Fees for physician services increasing at slower rate. *American Medical News* Feb 8, 1993, 16.
7. Anderson K: Health spending: An economic elixir. *USA Today* May 6, 1991, 3B.
8. Adelman S: Jobs: Hidden element in health care system. *American Medical News* Feb 1, 1993, 23.
9. Bennett I, Aron F: State of the profession. *Optom Econ* Oct 1992, 10.
10. Johnson J: Medicare Part B growth slumps in 1992. *American Medical News* Feb 15, 1993, 1.
11. Foreman J: Medicare trust funds on shaky grounds. *Arch Ophthalmol 1993;111:173.*
12. Mitchell JB, Wedig G, Cromwell J: The Medicare physician fee freeze: What really happened? *Health Aff (Millwood) 1989;8(1):21–33.*
13. Compiled by the American College of Surgeons from 1990 Medicare MBAD files.
14. Physician Payment Review Commission. *Annual Report to Congress* 1992, 4.
15 Iglehart JK: The American health care system. *N Engl J Med 1993; 328:896–900.*
16 Borzo G: Federal mandates not the cause of Medicaid cost explosion. *American Medical News* Feb 8, 1993, 11.
17. Gross S: Medicaid bill for state to rise $213 million. *St. Louis Business Journal* (get date).
18. Clemets M: Health care premiums to surge again. *St. Louis Business Journal* Jan 11–17, 1993, 1.
19. Larkin H: Higher benefits costs bring headaches to doctors. *American Medical News* Feb 24, 1993, 13–14.
20. Maynard M: GM white collar workers lose free health. *USA Today* Aug 26, 1992, B1.
21. Levin D: GM lost $23.3 billion last year. *The New York Times* Feb 12,

CHAPTER 1
ETHICS

CHAPTER 2
THE COSTS OF
HEALTH CARE

1993, C1.

22. White J: GM is headed for clash with workers over reductions in jobs, health benefits. *The Wall Street Journal* Aug 24, 1992, A3.

23. Kramon G: Business and health: Two companies cut medical costs. *The New York Times* Nov 7, 1989, 26.

24. Freudenheim M: The Xerox health care model. *The New York Times* Feb 13, 1993, C1.

25. Steinmetz G: States take on the job of holding down medical costs of Workers' Compensation. *The Wall Street Journal* Mar 4, 1993, B1.

26. Kerr P: The high cost of job injury claims. *The New York Times* Feb 22, 1993, C1.

27. Freudenheim M: Unions joining discount plan. *The New York Times* Aug 14, 1990, C2.

28. Crenshaw AB: Rising costs of benefits may hold down wages. *The Washington Post* Jul 12, 1991, GET.

29. Iglehart JK: The American health care system—private insurance. *N Engl J Med 1992;326:1715–1720.*

30. American Medical Association: *Policy research perspectives: The burden of health benefits on American business.* Center for Health Policy Research, Jul 10, 1992.

31. Rose R: Firms' attempts to cut health care benefits break calm of retirement. *The Wall Street Journal* Feb 24, 1993, A1.

32. Hemenway D, Killen A, Cashman SR, et al: Physician responses to financial incentives. *N Engl J Med 1990;332:1059–1063.*

33. Hillman BJ, Olson GT, Griffith PE, et al: Physicians' utilization and charges for outpatient diagnostic imaging in a Medicare population. *JAMA 1992;268:2050–2054.*

34. Gianelli DM: Stark seeks stiffer self-referral standards. *American Medical News* Jan 25, 1993, 3.

35. Conflicts of interest: Physician ownership of medical facilities. *JAMA 1992;267:2366–2369.*

36. Leape L, Hilborne LH, Park RE, et al: The appropriateness of use of coronary artery bypass graft surgery in New York state. *JAMA 1993; 269:753–760.*

37. Hilborne LH, Leape LL, Bernstein SJ, et al: The appropriateness of use of percutaneous transluminal coronary angioplasty in New York state. *JAMA 1993;269:761–765.*

38. Bernstein SJ, Hilborne LH, Leape LL, et al: The appropriateness of use of coronary angiography in New York state. *JAMA 1993;269:766–769.*

39. Eisenberg DM, Kessler RC, Foster C, et al: Unconventional medicine in the United States: Prevalence, costs, and patterns of use. *N Engl J Med 1993;328;246–252.*

40. Manago M: *Statement for the Subcommittee on Health, House Ways and Means Committee on Medicare Fraud, Waste and Abuse.* Washington, DC: Government Printing Office, Jun 14, 1990.

41. Gatty B: Patient benefits of cataract surgery high, say researchers. *Ophthalmology Times* Jul 15, 1990, 4.

42. Grumbach K, Lee PR: How many physicians can we afford? *JAMA 1991;265:2369–2370.*

43. Noreika JC: The oversupply of ophthalmic practitioners. *Am J Ophthalmol 1990;109:593–597.*

44. *Weighing the options for change in the '90s: Opportunities for ophthalmology.* American Acadamy of Ophthalmology (Environmental Analysis), San Francisco, 1991.

45. Total number of positions and first-year positions reported available for 1992. *JAMA 1992;268:1172.*

46. Ginsberg E: High-tech medicine and rising health care costs. *JAMA 1990;263:1820–1822.*

47. AMA/Specialty Society Medical Liability Project: Can we afford the cost of medical liability? Aug 1992.

48. McCormick B: Study: Defensive medicine costs nearly $10 billion. *American Medical News* Feb 15, 1993, 4.

49. American Medical Association. The costs of professional liability in the 1980s. Report of the Center for Health Policy Research, 1990.

50. Novack J: Someone else will pay. *Forbes* Mar 5, 1990, 93.
51. Usdansky ML: "Nation of youth" growing long in the tooth. *USA Today* Nov 10, 1992, 10A.
52. Schneider EL, Guralnik JM: The aging of America. Impact on health care costs. *JAMA 1990;263:2335–2340.*
53. Health Policy Briefs: Administrative Costs, American Medical Association, Group on Health Policy, Dec 1992.
54. Woolhandler S, Himmelstein DU: The deteriorating administrative efficiency of the US health care system. *N Engl J Med 1991;324:1253–1258.*
55. Thorpe KE: Inside the black box of administrative costs. *Health Aff (Millwood) 1992;11(2):41–55.*
56. Ruffenach G: Firms use financial incentives to make employees seek lower health-care costs. *The Wall Street Journal* Feb 9, 1993, B1.
57. Advocacy Briefs: US health spending compared with other countries. American Medical Association, Office of Policy Communication and Advocacy Support, Oct 1991.
58. Farrell C: Health care costs: Don't be too quick with the scalpel. *Business Week* Mar 15, 1993, 80.
59. Moyer ME: A revised look at the number of uninsured Americans. *Health Aff (Millwood) 1989;8(2):102–110.*
60. Blendon RJ, Donelan K: The public and the emerging debate over national health insurance. *N Engl J Med 1990;323:208–212.*
61. Advocacy Briefs: The impact of violence. American Medical Association, Office of Policy Communication and Advocacy Suport, Apr 1992.
62. Advocacy Briefs: Infant mortality. American Medical Association, Office of Policy Communication and Advocacy Support, Oct 1991.
63. U.S. health care: Patients have an Rx. *Medical Economics* Nov 16, 1992, 28.
64. Smith MD, Altman DE, Leitman R, et al: Taking the public's pulse on health system reform. *Health Aff (Millwood) 1992;11(2):125–133.*
65. Majority of Americans prefer to keep health insurance private. *Business and Health* Mar 1992, 10.
66. Cantor JC, Barrand NL, Desonia RA, et al: Business leaders' views on American health care. *Health Aff (Millwood) 1991;10(1):98–105.*
67. Employers will unite to push health reforms. *Medical Economics* Feb 22, 1993, 184.
68. Recipe for lower health costs: A dash of this, a drop of that.... *Medical Economics* Jun 3, 1991, 148.
69. Murray D: How sick is the system? *Medical Economics* Sep 21, 1992, 44–108.
70. Stout H, Wartzman R: White House considers taxes to cover health-care costs of up to $90 billion. *The Wall Street Journal* Feb 16, 1993.
71. Makinson L: Political contributions from the health and insurance industries. *Health Aff (Millwood) 1992;11(4):119–144.*
72. Angell M: The presidential candidates and health care reform. *N Engl J Med 1992;327:800–801.*
73. Rachlis M, Kushner C: What's really wrong with Canadian health care. *Medical Economics* Jul 6, 1992, 178–195.
74. Farnsworth CH: Now patients are paying amid Canadian cutbacks. *The New York Times* Mar 7, 1993, A1.
75. Canadian Health Insurance: Lessons for the United States. General Accounting Office, Report to the Chairman, Committee on Government Operations, House of Representatives, Jun 1991, 32–33.
76. Katz SJ, Mizgala HF, Welch HG: British Columbia sends patients to Seattle for coronary artery surgery: Bypassing the queue in Canada. *JAMA 1991;266:1108–1111.*
77. Iglehart JK: Health policy report: Germany's health care system. *N Engl J Med 1991;324:503–508.*
78. Stevens C: Does Germany hold the key to U.S. health care reform? *Medical Economics* Jan 6 1992, 148–156.
79. Meyer H: New health controls are approved in Germany. *American Medical News* Feb 15, 1993, 9.
80. Lister J: Reform of the British National Health Service: From white paper to bill in Parliament. *N Eng J Med 1990;322:410–412.*
81. Ikegami N: Japanese health care: Low cost through regulated fees.

Health Aff (Millwood) 1991;10(3):87–109.

82. Sterngold J: Japan's health care: Cradle, grave and no frills. *The New York Times* Dec 28, 1992, A1.

83. Eisenstodt G: The doctor's margin. *Forbes* Nov 23, 1992, 44–45.

84. Stout H: New concept for health care wins support. *The Wall Street Journal* Nov 2, 1992, B1.

85. Enthoven AC, Kronick R: Universal health insurance through incentives reform. *JAMA 1991;265:2532–2536.*

86. Anders G, Stout H: 'Managed competition' scores victory in California on health-care premiums. *The Wall Street Journal* Feb 11, 1993, B8.

87. Reinhold R: Wrestling health care costs to the mat. *The New York Times* Feb 10, 1993, A1.

88. Jones D: CEOs on the summit: Managed competition that works. *The Wall Street Journal* Dec 15, 1992, A18.

89. Winslow R: Employers' attack on health care costs spurs changes in Minnesota. *The Wall Street Journal* Feb 26, 1993, A1.

90. Maryland considers managed competition reform. *American Medical News* Feb 8, 1993, 20.

91. Johnsson J: Detroit doctors fear 'big 3' network may run over them. *American Medical News* Mar 15, 1993, 3.

92. Simmons HE, Rhoades MM, Goldberg MA: Comprehensive health care reform and managed competition. *N Engl J Med 1992;327:1525–1528.*

93. Relman A: Controlling costs by "managed competition"—would it work? *N Engl J Med 1993;328:133–135.*

94. Kronick R, Goodman DC, Wennberg J: The marketplace in health care reform: The demographic limitations of managed competition. *N Engl J Med 1993;328:148–152.*

95. McNamee M: The flaws in a model health care system. *Business Week* Mar 15, 1993, 43.

96. Wartzman R, Stout H: After diagnosing a case of out-of-control-costs, health strategist magaziner now must find cure. *The Wall Street Journal* Mar 15, 1993, A12.

97. Foreman J: Health Access America revisited and revised. *Arch Ophthalmol 1992;110:1690.*

98. Access to health care: The American debate—"play or pay." The Principal Financial Group, ZZ4917.

99. Painter J: "Play or pay" approach to health system reform. American Medical Association, Report of the Board of Trustees (RR:A-92), 1992.

100. Vagelos PR: 'Pay or play': How to stifle medical progress. *The Wall Street Journal* Oct 20, 1992, A14.

101. Physicians for a National Health Program, Chicago, IL.

102. Brown ER: Health USA: A national program for the United States. *JAMA 1992;267:552–558.*

103. Van Buskirk EM: Managed glaucoma care. *J Glaucoma 1993;2:68–74.*

104. Ellwood P, Etheredge L: The 21st century American health system: Health care reform through managed competition. *The Jackson Hole Group Proposals* Sept 1991.

105. Rosenthal E: Insurers second-guess doctors, provoke debate over savings. *The New York Times* Jan 24, 1993, A1.

106. Iglehart JK: The American health care system: Managed care. *N Engl J Med 1992;327:742–747.*

107. Sullivan CB, Miller M, Feldman R, et al: Employer-sponsored health insurance in 1991. *Health Aff (Millwood) 1992;11(4):172–185.*

108. Johnson J: HMO industry expected to see growth in 1993. *American Medical News* Dec 28, 1992, 14.

109. Murray D: Managed care: The payoff keeps getting better. *Medical Economics* Dec 7, 1992, 124–142.

110. Pokalo CL: Can you manage managed care? *Ocular Surgery News* Jan 1, 1993, 10.

111. Whitfield L, Grimes G: *Eye physicians file suit to stop federal Medicare cataract test program.* American Acadamy of Ophthalmology (News Release), San Francisco, May 1, 1991.

112. Pokalo CL: Demonstration sites named; bids revealed. *Ocular Surgery News* Feb 15, 1993, 3.

113. Insurance companies in ten states offer managed care plan for Medicare patients. *Ocular Surgery News* Feb 15, 1993, 57.
114. Borzo G: States trying managed care now, rather than waiting for reform. *American Medical News* Feb 8, 1993, 2.
115. Moon M, Holahan J: Can states take the lead in health care reform? *JAMA 1992;268:1500–1594.*
116. Somerville J: Oregon waiver opens way for state reform experiments. *American Medical News* Apr 5, 1993.
117. Hsiao WC, Braun P, Dunn D, et al: Resource-based relative values. An overview. *JAMA 1988;260:2347–2353.*
118. Hsiao WC, Yntema DB, Braun P, et al: Measurement and analysis of intraservice work. *JAMA 1988;260:2361–2370.*
119. Iglehart JK: The new law on Medicare's payments to physicians. *N Engl J Med 1990;322:1247–1252.*
120. *Federal Register 1991;56(108):25792–25867.*
121. *Federal Register 1991;56(227):59502–59819.*
122. *Federal Register 1992;57(228):55897–56230.*
123. Proposed Medicare cuts could be deep and far reaching. *Argus* Mar 1993, 4.
124. *Ocular Surgery News* Feb 1, 1993, 39.
125. Todd JS: 1993 Medicare payment schedule. American Medical Association, Nov 25, 1992.
126. McIlrath S: Congress lets volume performance levels rise. *American Medical News* Dec 14, 1992, A1.
127. McIlrath S: Doctors' gain falls short of payment reform target. *American Medical News* Mar 15, 1993, A1.
128. McIlrath S: Cut Medicare to ease the deficit? *American Medical News* Mar 1, 1993, A1.
129. Pear R: Putting limits on the growth of Medicare. *The New York Times* Feb 18, 1993, A15.
130. McIlrath S: Participation rates up for Medicare despite RBRVS. *American Medical News* Apr 13, 1992, A1.
131. McMenamin P: Personal communication, 1990.
132. Goldberg JH: Ophthalmologists' earnings shrink. *Medical Economics* Apr 12, 1993, 83–96.
133. *The Physician's Advisor 1992;92(11):1.*

 1. Hatlie MJ: Professional liability: The case for federal reform. *JAMA 1990;263:584–586.*
 2. Torry K: Drop in premiums predicted to be short-term situation. *American Medical News* Jan 8, 1990, 40.
 3. Tolchin M: Concern over the costs of malpractice liability. *The New York Times* Nov 5, 1989, E4.
 4. Stodghill R: Is this liability law a gravy train? *Business Week* Nov 6, 1989, 93–94.
 5. Mahoney RJ, Littlejohn SE: Lawsuits becoming a liability for nation. *The St. Louis Post Dispatch* Jan 3, 1990, Op-ed.
 6. Marcus AD: Juries rule against "tort reform" with huge awards. *The Wall Street Journal* Feb 9, 1990, B1.
 7. Brennan TA, Leape LL, Laird NM, et al: Incidence of adverse events and negligence in hospitalized patients. *N Engl J Med 1991;324:370–376.*
 8. Smith HE: The incidence of liability claims in ophthalmology as compared with other specialties. *Ophthalmology 1990;97:1376–1378.*
 9. Insler MS: Louisiana's medical review panel. *Surv Ophthalmol 1989;34:204–208.*
10. Bettman JE: Seven hundred medicolegal cases in ophthalmology. *Ophthalmology 1990;97:1379–1384.*
11. *Professional Liability Issues in Ophthalmology.* OMIC Risk Management Seminar, Chicago, Jun 25, 1992.
12. Johnson KB, Hirshfeld EB, Ile ML, et al: *Legal Implications of Practice Parameters,* Vol. 2. Chicago: American Medical Association, 1990.
13. *The Risk Controller,* Vol. 2. Newsletter, Risk Control Associates, Nov 1989.
14. Rein H: *Ocular Surgery News* Aug 1, 1989, 32.

CHAPTER 3
RISK MANAGEMENT AND MALPRACTICE

15. Foreman J: Medical liability tort reform receives congressional attention. *Arch Ophthalmol 1990;108:490.*
16. Freudenheim M: Limiting awards in malpractice. *The New York Times* Mar 19,1991, C2.
17. Burkhart J (ed): How the National Practitioner Data Bank can affect you. *JAMA 1991;265:2239.*
18. Johnson ID: Reports to the National Practioner Data Bank. *JAMA 1991;265:407–411.*
19. O'Day D: A new guideline for patients with cataract. *Arch Ophthalmol 1993;111:317–318.*
20. McIntyre DJ: *Guidelines for Cataract Practice.* Bellevue, WA, Feb 18, 1993.
21. Risk Control Associates data.
22. Golin CB: Buying tail coverage: Will the burden lighten? *J Med Pract Manag 1990;5:175–178.*
23. AMA/Specialty Society Medical Liability Project: *Risk Management Principles and Commentaries for the Medical Office.* Chicago: American Medical Association, 1990.
24. Board of Directors: *Risk Management Guidelines for Ophthalmologists' Staff.* San Francisco: American Academy of Ophthalmology, 1989.
25. Hepler RS: Ophthalmology personnel in risk management. *Ophthalmology 1990;97:1385–1387.*
26. *The Malpractice Suit: A Survival Guide for Physicians and Their Families.* Watertown, MA: Eidetics.
27 Board of Directors: *Expert Testimony By Ophthalmologists KB-PS28-89.* San Francisco: American Academy of Ophthalmology, 1989.
28. Anderson B Jr: The expert witness. *Ophthalmology 1990;97:1390–1391.*

CHAPTER 4
STARTING AND DEVELOPING A PRACTICE

1. Landau RJ: Be specific, reasonable in drafting employee "No Complete" clause. *Ophthalmology Times* May 1, 1990, 15.
2. Gerber PC: What can you learn from the Japanese? *Ophthalmology Times* Dec 1, 1992, 17–20.
3. Rudy PH: Avoiding wrongful termination and discrimination suits through updated policies. Presented at the Vail Management Institute, Dec 22, 1992.
4. Lawlor J: Contractors help firms save money. *USA Today* Mar 3, 1993, B1.
5. Deane LN: Know the tax difference between employees and independent contractors. *Ophthalmology Times* Mar 15, 1992, 22–23.
6. Goldberg MA: Hiring decisions that could incite IRS scrutiny. *Medical Economics* Mar 22, 1993, 54–57.
7. Rudy P: Doing a legal audit of your organization. Presented at the Vail Management Institute, Dec 22, 1992.
8. *Federal Register, 1991;56(235): 64175–64182.*
9. Harr D: OSHA rules on bloodborne pathogens apply to your ophthalmology practice. *Ocular Surgery News* Sep 1, 1992, 12.
10. Adler A: Blood and body fluid exposures. Presented at the Vail Management Institute, Dec 23, 1992.
11. Fleming SH: OSHA bloodborne pathogens final standard. *Metropolitan Medicine* May 1992, 22–23.
12. Americans with Disabilities Act: What you need to know for your office accomodations and employment policies. *Argus* Jul 1992, 16.
13. Gerber PC: The Americans with Disabilities Act. *Ophthalmology Management* Jan 1, 1993, 15–18.
14. The Americans with Disabilities Act: A prescription for compliance. *American Medical Association* Oct 1992.
15. Frum D, Brennan J: Oh my aching...you name it. *Forbes* Apr 26, 1993, 52–54.
16. Janofsky J: Whoever wrote the ADA regs never ran a business. *The Wall Street Journal* Mar 15, 1993, A12.
17. Clinton Signs FLMA, *Labor and Employment Legislative Watch.* Peper, Martin, Jensen, Maichel and Hetlage, Attorneys at Law. Spring, 1993.
18. *Federal Register 1991;56(145)35953–35987.*
19. Relman A: What market values are doing to medicine. *The Atlantic*

Monthly Mar 1992, 99–106.

20. Relman AS: "Self Referral"—What's at stake. *N Eng J Med 1992;327:1322–1524.*

21. Tenery RM: Should physicians abide by a higher standard? *American Medical News* Feb 8, 1993, 25.

22. Todd JS: Must the law assure ethical behavior? *JAMA 1992;268:98.*

23. Mitchell JM, Scott ES: New evidence of the prevalence and scope of physician joint services. *JAMA 1992;267:80–82.*

24. Hillman BJ, Olson GT, Griffith P, et al: Physician utilization and charges for outpatient diagnostic imaging in a Medicare population. *JAMA 1992;268:2050–2054.*

25. Mitchell JM, Scott E: Physician ownership of physical therapy services: Effects on charges, utilization, profits, and service characteristics. *JAMA 1992;268:2055–2059.*

26. Mitchell JM, Sunshine JH: Consequences of physicians' ownership of health care facilities—joint ventures in radiation therapy. *N Engl J Med 1992;327:1497–1501.*

27. Swedlow A, Johnson G, Smithline N, et al: Increased costs and rates of use in the California Workers' Compensation system as a result of self referral by physicians. *N Engl J Med 1992;327:1502–1506.*

28. Conflicts of interest: Physician ownership of medical facilities. *JAMA 1992;267:2366–2369.*

29. Gianelli DM: Stark seeks stiffer self-referral standards. *American Medical News* Jan 25, 1993, 3.

1. Advantages and disadvantages to managed care eye care plans. *Argus* March 1993; 21–22.

2. Handling managed care in a successful practice. *The Physician's Advisory,* special report, June 1993; 1–8.

3. Anders GT: Managed care contracts: Evaluating the financial returns. *The Health Care Group Forecast* Spring 1993; 2.

4. Holoweiko M: Don't get squeezed by a managed-care contract. *Medical Economics* July 22, 1991; 106–113.

5. Holoweiko M: How managed care contracts can drag down your income. *Medical Economics* August 5, 1991; 95–102.

6. Weber G: Capitation: A guide to end the confusion. *Argus* June 1993; 19.

7. The informed practitioner: Contracting with managed care plans. *Medical Practice Management, Management Briefs* 1993; 8(4):242.

8. Choosing a managed care plan: Tips on how to evaluate what will work for you. *Argus* March 1993; 23.

9. Gallagher J: Trends in managed care contracting. *The Medical Staff Counselor* 1991; 5:11–16.

10. Stromberg RE, Bowman AK: Hold harmless clauses may increase physician's liability. *Ophthalmic Risk Management Digest* Spring 1993; 5.

11. *Ophthalmology Software Directory and Buyers' Guide,* Vol 3, No 1, Spring 1993.

12. CPT 1992. *American Medical Association,* Chicago, 1991.

13. *Federal Register 1991;56(227):59529.*

14. Chriss I: Medicare as secondary payer: Mastering the maze. *Argus* January 1993; 16.

CHAPTER 5
PRACTICE CASH
FLOW MANAGEMENT

RECOMMENDED READINGS

1. Byron HM, Maller BS, Meltzer GE: *Future Focus: Ophthalmology Career Management.* Irvine, CA, SEE Inc., 1989.

   Written by two practicing ophthalmologists and an experienced practice management advisor, this book is geared to residents and new practitioners and is the text for a series of seminars presented throughout the country. It is ophthalmology specific, quite detailed, and deals with personal goal setting as well as other topics. There is a good section on buy-ins and contracts.

2. Farber L (ed): *Encyclopedia of Practice and Financial Management.* Oradel, NJ, Medical Economics, 1985.

   A true encyclopedia of practice management ideas that covers every important aspect in detail. Not all ideas are germane to ophthalmology. There is also an excellent section on personal financial management.

3. Ophthstart-Guidelines: *Selecting and Starting a Practice in Ophthalmology.* Oradel, NJ, Medical Economics, 1988.

   Similar to *Future Focus.* It is a bit more "nuts-and-bolts," and also serves as the text for practice management seminars held across the country for residents.

4. *The Guide. A Handbook to Building and Maintaining a Successful Ophthalmic Practice.* San Francisco, American Academy of Ophthalmology.

   An ongoing modular series covering personnel, office management, office finance, and retirement (which includes buy-in and buy-out arrangements). Additional sections on marketing insurance and dispensing are planned. All were developed through the Practice Management Committee and have been well received. They are ophthalmology specific and contain many practical hints for both general ophthalmologists and subspecialists.

5. Wold CR (ed): *Managing Your Medical Practice.* New York, Matthew Bender, 1991.

   A loose-leaf book whose modular format lends itself to timely updates (the most recent is on CPT-ICD-9 coding). Does not deal with personal financial planning in any detail.

INDEX

CUMULATIVE INDEX, VOLS. 1–10

PRACTICE MANAGEMENT

PRACTICE MANAGEMENT